The Business of Private Medical Practice

RAY STANBRIDGE

RADCLIFFE MEDICAL PRESS

© 1999 Ray Stanbridge

Radcliffe Medical Press Ltd
18 Marcham Road, Abingdon, Oxon OX14 1AA

British Library Cataloguing in Publication Data

A catalogue record for this book is availabe from the British Library.

ISBN 1 85775 223 6

Typeset by Action Publishing Technology, Gloucester

Contents

Preface

A significant number of British medical consultants' private practice businesses are larger, in turnover terms, than many so-called small businesses, such as farms, retail shops, manufacturing, haulage and even firms of accountants and solicitors. Many of these latter businesses have access to, and do use, a vast array of help provided by the State, local authorities, local Training and Education Councils, academics and others. Much has also been written to advise these businesses on how to grow and develop.

Yet strangely little has been done to assist medical consultants in their approach to and management of their businesses. Medical courses generally lack business training, and professional bodies do not seem to rank business matters as taking a priority in post-qualification education programmes.

Most medical consultants with a private practice have stumbled into a business education and learnt by their mistakes. Whether it be for professional jealousy or other reasons, consultants are reluctant to impart their business knowledge and experiences to colleagues. Every consultant, it seems, has to commence their business life with a standing start. As a practising accountant, it is clear that there are common themes that do characterise the more successful private practices. This book draws on some of these themes to provide a basis for business conduct and management for those consultants new to business, and for those who have some experience. It reports on some of the 'secrets' of the successful business professional.

Perhaps not unsurprisingly, even those financially successful clients of my own business are unwilling to write a foreword, for fear of releasing individual secrets to their competitors! It is therefore left to me to hope that the reader will find something in this text to help improve the management of his or her medical consultancy business. It is hoped that, in time, the reader will create secrets of their own as to their business success!

Ray Stanbridge
October 1998

Acknowledgements

I am indebted to all my clients in private medical practice who have taught me far more about their businesses than I ever thought there was to know. The contribution of Dr Alan Bailey to the thoughts on medical insurance companies in Chapter 10 is acknowledged with gratitude. My particular thanks are due to Mrs Andrea Butler who has managed to make sense of my notes and thoughts.

This book is dedicated to my three children, Tim, Nicola and Felicity.

1

The business of private practice: an overview

Private medical practice in the United Kingdom is a significant industry, worth about £652 million in 1996, according to research.[1] There are an estimated 17 500 medically qualified individuals engaged in private practice, each earning, therefore, an average of £37 000 in gross fees. These bland figures do not in any way describe the diversity of the industry and the significant variation in growth and financial performance of individual businesses.

The industry consists of start-up businesses, such as those established by newly qualified consultants; mature businesses; and declining businesses, owned and managed by those who are close to retirement, or who have, for whatever reason, lost their interest in private practice. It consists of full-time, part-time, casual and very occasional businesses. Individual private practice proprietors range from those with classic economic objectives, in terms of profit maximisation, to those who find the concept of private practice political anathema. The goals of business owners vary enormously. There are those who are looking for private practice as a small adjunct to their NHS salaries to provide, for example, for their children's education or for holidays. Others wish to create

[1] Laing Buisson (1998) *Laing's Review of Private Healthcare*. Laing Buisson, London.

a profitable asset which they can sell and, in extreme examples, can possibly seek to float publicly.

The range of the structure of individual private practice businesses and the objectives of their proprietors is enormous, both absolutely and relatively. In addition, structures and objectives do change with time and individual businesses can generate a life of their own. In this respect, the private medical practice shows no different characteristics to those exhibited by the mass of private businesses in the UK.

Is there a future for private practice?

There is evidence in the marketplace that, I believe, is favourable towards the future growth and prosperity of private practice in the UK.

First, the NHS, the mainstream of the country's health service for some 50 years, is showing signs of severe financial exhaustion. Many medical practitioners see this on a daily basis, in the form of increased waiting lists, cuts in services, rationing of non-essential services and the shutting down or hibernation of established hospital departments. Despite recent Government promises for more assistance, the UK is discovering that it cannot support, financially, a totally comprehensive and free medical service.

Second, the General Medical Council (GMC) is realising that the market is changing and has moved, in recent years, to partially help the industry. For example, it is probably likely to lift the ban on the advertising and marketing of services by specialists over the next few years. Such a step is entirely logical as GPs have been allowed to advertise since 1990. Many consultants in practice already market their services, and such a change in ruling will only rationalise what is happening in the marketplace. By its own comments, the GMC suggests that it cannot police and restrain fundamental market changes.

Third, the climate of competition has spread to the medical insurance industry, which is now regularly able to introduce new product designs to widen its market share and to open up markets.

These three factors will, I believe, open up the future market for private practice. It is not difficult to see that a fundamental and ongoing cash crisis in the NHS will result, at some point, in a political decision to reduce further the service to accident and emergency departments and to encourage individuals to take out private insurance for their medical protection. The potential removal of GMC restrictions will encourage medical practices to utilise the skills of business management and marketing. The increasing influence of medical insurance companies with their own dedicated network of hospitals may mean that they, rather than the NHS, will become the employers of the future.

The need for improved business management

Economic changes in the market will, in time, result in changes in the training and management of those entering and enjoying the benefits of private practice. In future years, those choosing this path as their primary source of income will need to become businessmen or women. They will require marketing, financial management, time management, negotiating and personnel skills. They will need to build a team of professional advisors, including accountants, lawyers and, I suspect, public relations and marketing specialists. Given the economic changes that are taking place, together with the introduction of the new 'self assessment' tax regime from 1996/97, financial management will become an increasingly important feature of even the smallest private practice. In addition, medical practitioners in private practice will need to acquire and maintain the grit and determination necessary to succeed as small businessmen or women. Repeated evidence shows that in an ever-competitive market it is these skills, together with an element of ruthlessness, that differentiates between those who survive and those who fail.

In the future private medical marketplace there will be winners and losers. Choice of specialty and an understanding of location economics will be important. Those specialising in medical skills where the market has an ability to pay, will be better off than those who specialise in other areas. In simple terms, those who have an economic ability to pay are generally between the ages of 25 and 65. Location of private practice will also be important for business and financial success. There are geographical areas of the country with a greater ability to pay than others. But demographic patterns do change, and flexibility of location may also become an important feature.

Those who are able to acquire and use the business skills identified above will undoubtedly survive and prosper in the harsher, more competitive market ahead. Those who do not acquire the necessary business skills will undoubtedly wilt and fail. Those who choose to ignore the challenge of private practice will, in my view, remain paid employees of insurance companies or, in the longer term, of a restricted and refocused NHS. In the longer term, their incomes will in real terms remain static or even fall. Profits are generated primarily for the benefit of shareholders, and ongoing financial vigilance will be required in the NHS.

Will you succeed in private practice?

Observations made over the years and examination and review of numerous sets of accounts suggests that there are recognisable and distinct patterns relating to income growth and financial success from private practice. There is also a series of individual characteristics that appear to differentiate those who are, or eventually will become, established and financially profitable and those to whom private practice is, or will be, no more than a sideline.

The rise and fall of private practice performance is a continuum, and a number of basic 'rules' appears to govern progress. Rules are, of course, always made to be broken and there are many exceptions. Nevertheless, the rules of private practice are supported by at least some empirical evidence.

RULE 1: A consultant's earnings' growth is predictable
I have written above about the theory of the rise and fall of a private practice. The progress of a business can be characterised by an 'S' shaped pattern of growth and decline over time, as shown in Figure 1.1.

Stage 1 of a private practice is a slow rate of growth. Earnings typically remain low, and while there may be a great deal of

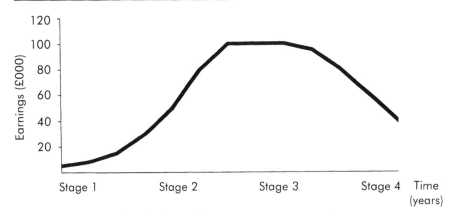

Figure 1.1 Model of medical consultants' private earnings cycle.

effort, this is not rewarded financially. Stage 2 represents a period of rapid growth in earnings and activity. At this stage all the hard work of stage 1 appears to be rewarded. Stage 3 represents the mature phase of the business. Earnings remain high but constant. The business has become part of the medical private sector establishment. Stage 4 represents the period of decline in the practice. This happens to all small and even large businesses. It comes about through changes in technology, customer or patient taste, increased competition or a change in motivation and effort on behalf of the proprietor.

In considering the position of a business, it is often helpful to determine at which stage it is. It is possible, of course, to try to influence the 'S' pattern and accelerate or decelerate its impact on personal lives and wealth.

RULE 2: Surgeons will earn more than physicians
The 'S' shaped curve is variable in both absolute and relative terms. With a few notable exceptions, the 'S' curve will show a higher level of earnings for surgeons rather than physicians. Ultimately this does reflect the market perception of the value of a surgeon's rather than a physician's services.

RULE 3: The first three years are critical
There is substantial accounting evidence to suggest that the first three years of private practice are critical in determining long-term

income levels from private practice. While there are, of course substantial variations, typical norms for private practice gross income for newly established consultants in 1997 before expenditure are shown in the table below.

Year following establishment of private practice	£000	
	Consultant surgeons	Consultant physicians
1	6	3
2	20	12
3	50	25

The harsh evidence from the marketplace suggests that those new consultants whose private practice *gross* incomes are *substantially and consistently below* the indicators above are unlikely to earn considerable sums from their practices in future. Conversely, those whose earnings are substantially higher than the indicators above can expect a long and profitable period in private practice.

RULE 4: Earn while you are young
Increasingly the world belongs to young people. To a large extent in the medical profession there is a series of rapid changes in technology, organisation, method of practice and attitudes towards patients.

While a large number of middle-aged consultants and beyond do earn substantial sums from private practice, market evidence suggests that there is a loose correlation between relatively high private practice earnings at a young age and at an older age. Those who do not start earning young are less likely to do so in later years.

It is relevant to comment that many successful women consultants do tend to start later in life than their male colleagues. Their patterns of income growth need to be considered in relation to their child-rearing roles, which, in purely financial terms, can inhibit the ability to earn when young.

The 'S' shaped curve can be identified for most practices. For some, stage 2 is very pronounced and financially rewarding. For others it can be very weak and can merge with stage 3, giving a relatively low continuing level of earnings from private practices.

What then influences these practices which have strong (i.e. financially successful) as opposed to weak stage 2 features? First, and of absolute importance, it comes back to the individual. Venture capitalists have long since identified the four characteristics of a successful business: people, people, people and product. Successful medical consultants in financial terms are those who have a clear sense of purpose, an ability to relate to people, substantial energy, an element of ruthlessness and a willingness to put business above pleasure while they are building their careers.

The second requirement for success is that of abundance of technical skills. The market for medical services increasingly requires speed, financial efficiency and, if appropriate, niche skills and knowledge. Those not possessing any of these skills are less likely to exhibit rapid income growth than those who do.

'Networking' is the third principal factor differentiating the financially successful medical practitioner in private practice from his or her colleagues. The medical industry is not unique in that it is all about people and contacts. The successful private practitioner will have a wide range of GP, hospital, managerial and other contacts which he or she is able to utilise and work with commercially.

Finally, there is always the element of luck. In client meetings, I have often heard of consultants referring to their colleagues as being lucky. As with all walks of life, luck does exist, and some people are naturally lucky. However, the successful generally create their own luck and certainly identify potentially lucky opportunities.

The objectives of this book

Given the factors that influence success, I believe that with a certain amount of background knowledge it is possible to *reasonably* predict a consultant's future level of earnings from private practice. Some in private practice will succeed and others will not. With this knowledge, it is possible for an individual consultant to plan and, if appropriate, improve his lifestyle and financial performance perhaps a little more scientifically than many appear to do so. This book provides some advice to both improve, and at the same time to reduce the level of uncertainty in, performance.

Business training will be increasingly important to the success of a private practice in future. As a second objective this book assists aspiring, new and existing members of medical private practice to cope with the range of business demands that will increasingly be placed upon them. It covers in outline a range of financial, marketing, tax, personnel and other topics necessary for business success in private practice over the millennium years.

This book can be no more than a useful compendium of business tips and advice. Topics can only be covered in outline, and on particular matters, specialist advice from other qualified professionals is essential. The challenge for those in private practice to improve their performance has to be matched by the challenges to professional accountants, lawyers and others who service the profession. They too need to hone their specialist skills to provide an adequate service.

The book makes no attempt to deal with particular medical issues or, for example, rules of professional conduct or discipline. It is focused on the medical practice as a commercial business.

Written in a simple style the book is appropriate reading for the common room, the train and even at bedtime. It encompasses the whole spectrum of medical practitioners from aspiring trainees to those who already have a mature, successful practice. The book will have succeeded if such successful men or women in the industry can identify at least one thing that they are not already doing.

2

Practice business organisation

When establishing a private practice, an individual consultant needs to consider how he or she is going to operate legally. There are essentially three alternative choices:

- the sole trader
- the partnership with others
- the limited company.

The modus operandi can change over a business lifetime and should be the subject of constant review. There are advantages and disadvantages in each form of trading and the relative merits of these features to an individual will change over time.

The sole trader

The vast majority of new consultants choose to establish themselves on a sole trader or individual practice basis. This is a very simple method of business organisation, which can be achieved with a minimum of paperwork. An individual can decide to establish a consulting business at a moment's notice. Apart from notifying the Inland Revenue and the Department of Social Security there is little more that in practical organisational terms has to be done.

The advantages of the 'sole trader' type of business organisational arrangements are that:

- it is essentially very simple

- paperwork and establishment/legal operational costs are at a minimum

- it is a very flexible means of trading that does not preclude alternative organisational structures at a later stage. Individuals can open and close private practices very easily

- ongoing organisational and management costs are low

- in the event of business failure, there is little public evidence. Individuals can return to alternative occupations without the opprobrium of public comments.

There are also a number of disadvantages in the 'sole trader' methods of practice. Most notable is the potential income tax inflexibility. Sole medical practitioners are taxed at the standard rate of income tax, currently 23% on taxable earnings between £4301 and £27 100, and 40% thereafter.

In practical terms, tax planning is frequently restricted to seeking to secure maximum relief from personal pension schemes or retirement annuity contracts as prescribed by the Revenue. Other methods of business organisation do offer greater flexibility for tax planning.

Other principal disadvantages of the 'sole trader' type of business organisation for consultants are that:

- it is a lonely form of business organisation. Some of the more successful businesses result from the activities of a team who are able to inter-relate and to deal collectively with opportunities and problems

- it is a very vulnerable form of business organisation. Death terminates the business instantly. Of more significance, however, is permanent debilitating sickness, accident or injury, which have an immediate impact on the business. While insurances can be taken out to protect income, these are rarely sufficient to fully offset the potential losses

- it is a very restrictive form of business organisation. The growth of the business is linked to a single consultant's available time. This in turn is linked to his or her predetermined time commitments to the NHS

- intrinsically, there is a higher risk of failure. Time commitments, personality, pressure from being a sole trader and a reluctance to commit full time to the business ensure that its ongoing existence is highly vulnerable

- there is a high risk of business mistakes and error. The sole trader has to have a wide range, not only of technical but also business skills. They have to embark on the learning curve and are more prone to make mistakes, which can be financially very costly.

The partnership

The partnership is the most common form of business arrangement used by GPs. A partnership allows individuals to act autonomously, subject to the rules governing the relationships between partners.

While the market circumstances are very different for consultants from those in which the GP operates, the concept of partnership for specialists is growing. I believe that there will be significant further growth in this area. An increasing number of specialists, such as anaesthetists and pathologists, do now operate under partnership arrangements. There is a growing recognition of the advantages of partnerships among other specialists.

The principal advantages of the partnership form of business organisation for consultants are that:

- work is able to be managed efficiently. Partners are able to offer cover at all times for their private individual and/or hospitals clients

- profits of the partnership are able to be distributed fairly and equitably

- a partnership is able to offer additional negotiation strengths, whether it be with, for example, a hospital or an insurance company

- there are opportunities for greater collective marketing and development of new services

- individual members of a partnership who, for example, suffer illness or injury, may not necessarily be financially penalised. The greater collective strengths of a partnership can ensure that individual partners are afforded higher income protection security than may be the case for a sole trader.

The principal disadvantages of the partnership form of business organisation are that:

- there is 'joint and several' responsibility for actions. For example, if a consultant is successfully sued for negligence, all partners may, in theory, and under the terms of the 1890 Partnership Act be liable for damages. Clearly individual indemnity insurance and the precise working of a partnership deed may restrict collective responsibility. However, as a general feature, partners are dependent on each others actions

- there is a greater administrative requirement than for a sole trader business. Administration costs will generally be higher for a partnership than for a sole trader

- there may be greater tax complications. While partnerships have emerged from the transitional changes following the introduction of the self assessment tax system there are new rules in operation. In particular, partnership tax returns are now obligatory. In addition, Inland Revenue assessments for partnerships have been replaced by self assessments on individual taxpayers. Individual partners must now include their share of partnership profits in their individual self assessment

- consultants, as individuals, may find it hard to work together. A partnership with internal conflict, lack of leadership and poor general management is doomed to long term failure.

The partnership agreement

While partnerships may operate under the very general loose terms of the 1890 Partnership Act, a written partnership agreement is, in my view, essential as the modus operandi of a successful business. The British Medical Association (BMA) has drawn up a list of essential clauses to be included in GP agreements. While there may be more flexibility in requirements of a consultant partnership a number of items are essential:

- details of the partners
- nature of the business
- dates of commencement and termination
- capital
- professional ethics and conduct
- medical indemnity
- role of the partners
- the partnership administrator or Chairman
- the partnership accountant
- bank account
- partnership income
- partnership expenses
- profits and losses
- income protection policy
- staffing policy
- provisions for joining and retiring partners
- income tax arrangements and policy
- holidays, maternity and partnership leave
- absence and illness policy (approved and unapproved)
- disciplinary procedures
- termination of partnership.

Planning the partnership

The partnership form of business organisation, to be successful, does require significant input at the pre-planning stage. A poorly thought through partnership philosophy and structure will not achieve the obvious stated advantages. There are a number of basic steps.

STEP 1: Identify the rationale
A potential partnership between like-minded consultants must have a clear business objective, and must be established to meet a clear market need. The market need can often be established by use of the simple SWOT analytical technique. This is a business appraisal tool which seeks to identify the *strengths* of a business, its *weaknesses*, the *opportunities* available and the *threats* facing it. A rigorous analysis along these lines can usually eliminate, on market and business grounds, a poor partnership concept.

STEP 2: Plan in advance to maximise success
In this respect the partnership agreement is the bible. In addition, the establishment of sound operating and accounting systems is essential if the partnership is to operate successfully.

STEP 3: Formally define the management structure
Sadly, the management of the partnership is frequently not given the attention it deserves. A clear formal definition of the role of the administrator and of the partners is essential in advance to avoid rancour and disharmony.

STEP 4: Agree the finances
Formal discussion and agreement on the financial aspects of the business are essential. In particular, the negotiation of banking facilities and the treatment of tax matters are two areas that frequently cause dissent. In operating a clear financial policy, the preparation of an operating budget and the management of the partnership against that budget is generally a sufficient first step.

STEP 5: Maintain ongoing business planning
To be successful, a consultant partnership has to be commercially

alive. For example, consideration has to be given to the reaction of competitors; discussion needs to be ongoing as to any new services that can be offered; positions need to be agreed, and varied, in terms of negotiations with other medical professionals, hospitals and insurance companies. Placid partnerships, without substance or ongoing life, are generally doomed to failure.

STEP 6: Above all, timing is important
Market opportunities come and go, and the medical sector is not exempt in this respect. Like-minded potential partners may show interest in the concept. If this proves to be lukewarm, the partnership will not work. If there is interest and appreciation of the market need, the detailed research and a clear timetable of action will give the best possible start to a new form of business organisation to many individual consultants.

The limited company

There is considerable interest among many consultants in the concept of a limited company as a means through which to practice and to provide shared service facilities, such as accommodation or staff. Usually this is driven from an apparent desire to save tax. For 1998/99 the current small companies rate of corporation tax of 21% on the first £300 000 of profits, rising to 31% on profits in excess of £1.5 million, appears attractive against standard income tax rates of 23% and 40%.

The advantages of a limited company, in addition to potential tax savings and opportunities for more sophisticated tax planning are that:

- a company has an entity of its own. It is separate, legally, from its proprietors and therefore offers a flexible means of trading

- in theory, it offers the potential of limited liability to the proprietors. However, in practice, creditors, bankers and mortgagors of any company routinely seek personal guarantees from directors. The advantage is often illusory

- there are considerable marketing opportunities. A 'branded' image can be created, which in turn can enhance a sale possibility. In theory, it is easier to sell the assets and business of a company rather than those of a sole trader and partnership practice

- there may be greater tax advantages through employing a spouse through a company rather than through a sole trader or partnership. Other costs may be deducted for corporation tax purposes that are disallowed for a sole trader

- a company structure can allow for more efficient pension planning than is possible through a sole trader or partnership arrangement. This is through, for example, executive pension or self-administered pension plans. In some cases these advantages can be very considerable indeed.

The principal disadvantages of the company form of business organisation for a consultant are:

- there are very strict and serious obligations on a consultant as a director of a company. These are considered below

- there are significant statutory, filing and accounting obligations placed on the officials of a company. These are considered below

- some of the perceived taxation advantages may be spurious. For example, if a consultant pays himself or herself a salary through the company he or she will have to deduct income tax according to his or her PAYE coding. In addition, the company will have to pay Class I employers' national insurance. This is currently at 10% increasing to 12.2% from 1999/2000. In individual cases, the net tax burden may be higher

- company accounts may have to be audited if turnover exceeds £350 000 per annum. This will place a greater administrative burden on the business

- as indicated above, the potential advantages of 'limited liability' may be illusory

- the medical defence bodies have indicated that they cannot normally indemnify corporations against negligence and other professional claims. Insurance is limited to individuals.

The obligations of a consultant as a company director

In essence, these are no different from the obligations facing any other director. A director has to constantly ensure that he or she is 'fit to act' as a company director. For example:

- his or her company is under proper control, including compliance with the Companies Acts and other legislation. The director has to ensure that accounting records are properly kept and that annual accounts are prepared and filed

- his or her company operates an effective system of financial control, and that suppliers, crown departments and other creditors are properly dealt with

- he or she takes early corrective action (including where necessary financial advice) when the company shows signs of getting into financial difficulties

- he or she generally manages the business with responsibility and with adequate skill and care to meet the needs of creditors.

In the event that the company fails, the consultant, in his or her capacity as a director, may be subject to proceedings under the Company Directors Disqualification Act 1986. This Act consolidated all previous disqualification legislation and introduced tougher provisions directed at those involved in the failure of a company and whose conduct calls into question their fitness to be involved in the management of other companies.

Duties and responsibilities of a company director

In addition to a consultant needing to satisfy the 'fitness to act' criteria, as a director he or she becomes legally responsible for the preparation of financial statements in compliance with the various Companies Acts and for their filing. In particular, a director has legal responsibilities to:

- ensure that his or her company maintains proper accounting records

- prepare and file accounts with Companies House in approved format which give a 'true and fair' view of the state of the company's affairs at balance sheet date

- prevent and detect a fraud, other irregularities and errors

- prepare a directors' report for each financial year containing information specified in the Companies Act

- consider and approve accounts

- send a copy of the accounts and directors' report to every shareholder and debenture holder in the company

- ensure that the company's tax affairs are in order. In particular, there is a requirement to return corporation tax form CT200 and, if appropriate, form CT201 to the Revenue and to meet the obligations of the new 'pay and file' regulations

- determine whether or not the company requires an audit or is subject to the exemption provisions.

The list of statutory and 'fitness to act' requirements on company directors is daunting. This is particularly so for many medical consultants, who generally do not have the necessary business, legal or accounting skills as part of their professional training.

A decision for a consultant to establish a company needs to be taken in conjunction with other professional advisors. Their potential role in supporting a consultant's business is considered in Chapter 8.

In conclusion, a consultant establishing an operating business has a choice of three basic means of organisation – as a sole trader, as a partnership with others or as a limited company. Each of these forms of business relationship has advantages and disadvantages. Hybrid arrangements are possible. The pros and cons are dynamic and will change over time, as market conditions change and as a consultant's business goals or objectives adjust. Constant review is necessary to ensure the optimum and, for many consultants, the most tax efficient means of operating.

3

Practice staffing

Staff are probably the most important asset of any business. Nowhere is this as true as it is in the medical consultant sector, where businesses are generally small and staff are totally interdependent. A consultant's practice can be made or broken by his or her relationship with staff and, in turn, their relationship with patients.

Many consultants are unfamiliar with both legal and business matters in terms of their relationships with staff, and these weaknesses and irregularities can ultimately affect performance.

Employment or self-employment?

It is of paramount importance to the legal relationship between a consultant and his or her staff as to whether they are classified as 'employed' or 'self-employed'. This is true in all cases, but in particular in respect of NHS secretaries undertaking private work.

Many consultants in private practice employ a range of workers, for example, full- or part-time secretaries, research assistants, assistants in operations and nursing and other support staff. Historically, the means of paying these workers has frequently been to treat them as 'casual'. More recently, the Revenue has changed its attitude to such an approach. One of the first targets of the Government's 'Spend-to-Save' initiative, introduced in 1997 to stop tax evasion, is to seek to bring as many people into an employed status as they can. By defining workers as 'employed', income tax and class one national insurance contributions can be paid at source.

The Revenue has issued a series of guidelines to assist consultants and others to determine whether their 'workers' are in fact 'employed' or 'self-employed'. Some key tests are listed below.

TEST 1
Is the true intention of the relationship between the consultant and the worker to avoid paying income tax and national insurance?

TEST 2
Is there any personal relationship between the consultant and the worker?

TEST 3
Is there a long-term business relationship between a consultant and the worker. For example, are services provided over a short period or over a continuous timescale?

TEST 4
Is the worker entitled to benefits such as sick pay?

TEST 5
Is the basis of payment *similar* to that expected by those in full-time employment, i.e. weekly or monthly pay? Does the worker submit regular or irregular invoices, for example?

TEST 6
Does the consultant exercise full control over the workers' activities?

TEST 7
Can the consultant terminate the relationship with the worker without any claim for dismissal or compensation? For example, is there any threat of industrial tribunal proceedings in the relationship?

TEST 8
Does the worker risk any of his or her money in the business? For

example, is there a financial penalty for making errors? Are there any arrangements for joint venture funding?

TEST 9
Does the worker provide any of his or her own tools and/or medical equipment?

TEST 10
Can the worker substitute somebody else to do the work, i.e. is the relationship between the consultant and the worker personal to him or her, or, for example, can the provider of the service send somebody else?

TEST 11
Is there any incentive for the worker to benefit from personal efficiency? For example, are any productivity payments made?

Other things being equal, if a consultant, in considering the status of any individual worker answers 'yes' to tests 1–6 and 'no' to tests 7–11, that worker would almost certainly be deemed by the Revenue to be an employee. As a result, the Revenue would look to the consultant to deduct income tax and class one national insurance from salaries, wages and any other remuneration paid. If there are three or more 'yes' answers to tests 1–6 and two or more 'no' answers to tests 7–11 it would be very unwise for a consultant not to treat his or her worker as an employee. Other cases may be more marginal and, as in all cases where there is the slightest uncertainty, professional help should be sought.

It is important for a consultant to determine correctly a worker's status. The penalties for making errors are severe. For example, the Revenue can look to a consultant to meet income tax/national insurance contributions as if a worker was an employee paid net. The potential liability for error can be considerable.

The consultants' employees

The employment of staff by a consultant does carry responsibilities. In particular the statutory rights of employees have to be acknowledged, respected and acted upon. The law is constantly changing and being updated. Any problems in interpretation should always be referred to legal advisors. However, basic rights are listed as follows, these rights generally apply to all employees and are not necessarily fully comprehensive:

- the right to receive itemised pay statements
- the right to enjoy trade union membership
- the right to enjoy time off work for trade union activities and for the performance of public duties (for example, acting as a magistrate or as a juror)
- the right for time off for antenatal care
- the right for a protected period of notice for redundancy
- the right not to be discriminated against in employment on the grounds of sex, age and race
- the right to receive a written contract of employment within a specified period of time. A basic contract should cover items such as the names of the parties, the commencement date, a reference to the continuity of employment provisions, the job title, the normal hours of work, the holiday entitlement and holiday pay, the provision of sick pay, provision (or otherwise) of pensions and other benefits, and provisions as to notice. In addition, many solicitors would advise that attached to an employment contract should be details of a grievance and disciplinary procedure. Modern contracts of employment incorporating terms of up-to-date legislation are available from many legal firms and also from the BMA. Those who do not issue their employees with proper contracts are storing up future trouble
- the right to a minimum wage. Enforcing legislation has now been passed.

Other rights are available to employees on a 'time-served' basis. These include, for example, the right to return to work after absence due to pregnancy and maternity leave, the right to receive redundancy pay and the right to claim against a consultant for unfair dismissal.

Unfair dismissal

In this current litigious environment, a significant number of consultant employers are, at one time or another, likely to be threatened with industrial tribunal proceedings for breach of employment rights. This is in circumstances where, for whatever reason, staff are dismissed and/or their contract determined. Sadly, many consultants are ill-prepared for such proceedings because:

- they have failed to ensure that their employees' rights are fully protected

- they have failed to prepare and update the relevant paperwork

- they have failed to take professional legal advice at an early stage.

In the event of a consultant employer dismissing an employee who subsequently commences proceedings, he or she has to prove, conclusively, that the termination of an employment contract was not 'unfair'. The onus is very much on the employer to provide the burden of proof. If a dismissal is not to be regarded by an industrial tribunal as being unfair, the consultant must show that the reason falls within any of the five following categories:

- gross misconduct. For example, assault in the consultant's rooms, drunkenness or other similar behaviour

- incapacity to perform the work. There is a long procedure to be followed for those consultants who feel any of their employees are incompetent. Legal advice at an early stage is essential to ensure that these procedures are complied with

- redundancy. In the event of a reconstruction of a consultant's business

- a legal impediment to continuing that employment. For example, the long term jailing of an employee following criminal prosecution

- 'some other substantive reasons'. It should be noted that a consultant employer can be held to have 'dismissed' a member of staff if the employee walks out in circumstances where the consultant's behaviour is held to justify his or her doing so without notice. This is known as 'constructive dismissal'.

Payroll management

A consultant with employees has, legally, to operate a PAYE scheme. Income tax and national insurance have to be deducted from an employee's pay and accounted for to the Revenue, normally on a monthly basis. The Inland Revenue does issue starter packs to employers which describe, in detail, the nature and operation of the PAYE scheme. They also operate a useful helpline service for those with queries or problems. In addition, most accountants will have some expertise in this area.

As part of the Revenue controls of PAYE schemes, a consultant employer has to prepare each year for each employee forms P60, P11D (for those earning more than £8500 per annum) and form P9D. Form P60 records the earnings and tax/national insurance deducted and forms P11D and P9D record the 'benefits in kind' received. The consultant has a legal obligation to file these forms with the Revenue not later than 6 July following the conclusion of a 5 April tax year.

Historically, many consultants have been noticeably lax in their treatment of PAYE records and reporting of taxable benefits to staff. Changing legislation and the expanding net of national insurance have forced changes. In addition, the Revenue has intensified its performance of visits to employers to ensure compliance with PAYE regulations and reporting requirements. The costs of non-compliance can be very severe, and a consultant employer can now be fined if he or she is late in filing forms or they are in any way inaccurate.

In managing a consultant's payroll and staff benefits records there are a number of essential tips:

- a consultant needs to ensure that records are maintained to a high standard of accuracy

- documentation has to be dealt with and filed in a timely

manner. If the consultant has other priorities, it is essential to ensure that somebody does deal with this administration

- advice is taken on what benefits in kind are tax efficient. For example, staff Christmas parties, subject to certain limits, do not attract tax. Similarly, costs of travel from work to home on occasional late nights will not normally attract a tax charge

- specialist tax advice is often beneficial to determine whether it is worth paying for an employee's private travel costs or fuel. This appears to be increasingly tax disadvantageous under the 1998 budget statement

- ensure, in particular, that very detailed and accurate records are maintained of an employee's business mileage. Systems need to be in place to ensure that these key pieces of data are readily available

- if staff do travel to work consider providing interest-free loans to employees for season-ticket travel. Currently there is no tax on loans to staff if the balance does not exceed £5000

- above all, maintain accurate records.

Statutory sick pay (SSP)

Employees working for a consultant are generally entitled to receive SSP from their employers for up to 28 weeks of sickness absence. SSP is paid at a flat weekly rate of £57.70 from 6 April 1998 and will usually be paid on an employee's normal pay day. In most cases, 87% of this cost can be recovered against regular national insurance contributions. The administration of SSP is highly complex and the Department of Social Security requires the maintenance of very detailed records. There are also very strict rules as to the *precise* eligibility of staff for payment of SSP. The reality is that for most consultants, the cost of preparing paperwork may be greater than the financial benefit to the employee.

From 6 April 1998, consultant employers can elect to 'opt out' of the SSP scheme, if they pay wages or salaries above the SSP rate of

£57.70 per week. Payments can be treated as if they were part of SSP and recovered accordingly. Given the small number of employees working in the majority of consultant practices, and the heavy paper load involved, this course is recommended. As a result, an element of the costs of maintenance for sick employees can be recovered against national insurance, and in some cases PAYE, without the detailed management required for a full SSP system.

Despite this general comment, detailed advice is necessary for most consultants to ensure compliance with the strict Social Security laws, and to ensure that maximum recovery is made against national insurance/taxation with minimum paperwork.

Statutory maternity pay (SMP)

All female employees are, in theory, liable to receive SMP when they are pregnant. SMP is payable currently at two rates over an 18-week period. The higher rate payment is based on 90% of an employee's earnings for the first six weeks and the lower rate at the flat rate of £57.70 from 6 April 1998 for the remaining 12 weeks. SMP is only available to employed staff who have worked for a consultant for at least 26 weeks. It is paid even if an employee is not returning to work.

Under the so-called 'small employers' relief', the vast majority of consultant employers will be able to recover 100% of SMP payments made, plus a further 6.5% through deductions from PAYE/NI liability. As with SSP, detailed records have to be maintained, which are subject to scrutiny from the Department of Social Security. In addition, strict adherence has to be made to the complex set of rules.

While this is very burdensome, given the rate at which SMP is paid for the first six weeks, there is at least some opportunity for overall tax savings for those consultants who employ their wives and can plan the dates of birth of their children reasonably accurately.

Employment of the wife or husband in the practice

There are often significant tax savings to be made for a consultant in private practice to employ his or her spouse in the business. Family tax savings of between £1000 and £1500 per annum are not uncommon through such a strategy, if two simple rules are followed.

The immediate, and obvious, first rule is that a spouse has to make an actual contribution to the business. Ever vigilant tax inspectors can and do argue that a spouse's costs are not 'wholly, necessarily and exclusively' incurred for the purpose of the practice. As a result, spouse costs can be disallowed in whole or in part against profit for tax purposes.

Second, under the self assessment tax rules, responsibility for assessing a spouse's business role is passed in the first instance back to the consultant. A series of simple steps will ensure maximum compliance with the rules:

- formally write down the work the spouse actually undertakes or will undertake in future. Prepare a job description

- take a view as to the market cost of employing an external party to undertake work. For example, what would be the actual cost to a consultant of employing somebody to deal with telephone messages, book-keeping and patient liaison/management. Such a 'market cost' provides a good guide as to what a spouse can actually be paid

- provide evidence of employment. It is particularly recommended that a spouse has a proper job description and a written contract of employment

- ensure that payments are made to the spouse in accordance with the contract of employment. It is surprising that many consultants still do not actually pay over monies claimed against their profits to their spouses. One of these key arguments is therefore instantly lost in any negotiation with the Revenue.

- operate the PAYE system properly

- maintain records in a disciplined manner.

If the management of a spouse's employment is in order, there will be immediate taxation savings to the family. In addition, the employment of a spouse in the business can generate opportunities for further tax saving. For example, a pension scheme can be established for a spouse; benefits may be provided on a tax efficient basis; and claims for use of domestic accommodation for business purposes may be enhanced and better argued. In addition, if partners are married, and both have medical qualifications, employment in the consultant's business can offer further opportunities for long-term tax planning between husband and wife.

Managing staff

In recent years, increasing attention has been given to the concept of 'total quality management' and 'customer care'. Customers have been recognised by businesses as being of paramount importance to their success. Substantial literature has been written and scores of business consultants now market advice on how to treat customers and to improve customer care. In reality, much of what is said is common sense.

Surgeons, physicians and others in private medical practice are in a market environment and have to compete with one another on a more discerning patient base, whether they operate wholly or partially in the private sector, the semi-privatised trusts or in the traditional NHS. They have increasingly to offer a high quality of efficient, competitive service with high standards of quality control and customer care.

In conveying their market image to patients, consultants have to rely on themselves and their staff. Managing staff to achieve maximum performance is a skill many lack. Those who manage and motivate their own staff well will achieve a better business performance.

While it is extremely difficult to advise on precisely how staff can be managed well, it is far easier to identify areas in which consultants have managed staff badly, to the detriment of their businesses. Some of the basic errors are listed below in somewhat of a light-hearted manner.

ERROR 1   Be mean with wages
While the medical secretary and assistant market is by no means unionised, there is a strong informal network. Secretaries have a good information network and are well able to identify where the best rates of pay can be earned for both full- and part-time work. Practice staff are economic animals and the best tend to gravitate towards the best payers. Those consultants who consistently underpay the market rate are generally rewarded with poorer quality staff, a higher turnover of staff, a less enthusiastic staff and more patient problems.

ERROR 2   Avoid capital expenditure
The office is changing rapidly and technology is taking over many of the more menial and repetitive office tasks. Many consultants are surprisingly ignorant of office technology and are reluctant to equip their offices with up-to-date equipment. Word processors, fax machines, modems, the Internet and integral computer systems are now a well-established part of any modern office. Those consultants who do invest in office technology at a level at least commensurate within their practice activity will be rewarded with a better quality of staff.

ERROR 3   Maintain a schedule of unplanned and irregular hours
The very nature of a consultant's business means that irregular hours have to be worked. Secretaries and practice staff do understand this. However, there are consultants who have no concept of planning their work hours, whether these be social or anti-social. Staff who have to cope with a total lack of time planning will not stay. Anti-social hours are not a 'turn off' for practice staff. Total lack of time planning is.

ERROR 4   Discourage training
The business world continues to change at a rapid pace. New technologies today are commonplace tomorrow. The growth of information technology and the pressure that this puts on all in business necessitates a constant programme of staff training. There are a large number of courses on offer for staff at all levels. Those consultants who encourage their staff to be up to date with technology and therefore able to manage it, will

have far more efficient businesses than those adopting a Luddite attitude.

ERROR 5   Maintain a poor consulting rooms environment
The varying standards of office accommodation, consulting rooms and general business ambience are extreme. The more sophisticated consultant practice makes full allowance for sensible secretarial and support staff space. Attention is given to furniture, lighting and decoration. Other practices operate from poor, cramped conditions with old and inappropriate furniture, and a Dickensian standard of lighting. Consultants who are able to offer a more attractive working environment will be sought out by better quality staff and patients.

ERROR 6   Let the boyfriend/girfriend visit regularly
Consultants show varying degrees of interest in the appearance of their waiting areas and who uses them. For example, the heavy-smoking, loud boyfriend of the practice secretary is not a sight that the majority of patients, who are commonly nervous and anxious, want to see in the waiting room.

ERROR 7   Ignore telephone manners
In most medical practices the interface between patient and the consultant is the secretary. He or she will make appointments, often notify results and act as a scrutiniser of further treatment. Those practices that employ secretarial staff with aggressive and abrupt telephone manners, a poor telephone voice or an apparent lack of understanding manner lose patients. The more successful practices generally employ sympathetic secretarial staff with efficient and caring telephone manners. Such staff reap economic dividends. Telephone training for those who have only basic skills frequently generates significant benefits and customer goodwill to the practice.

ERROR 8   Be mean with holidays
Staff working in medical practices are aware of the 'market rate' for holidays. Those consultants who do not recognise market conditions will encourage resentful staff and, in consequence, an underperforming business.

ERROR 9   Maintain a disorganised approach to accounting
The standards of consultants' books and records in the UK vary considerably. Some practice secretaries or book-keepers are compelled to try to maintain accounting records with a thoroughly disorganised boss. Poor invoicing, lack of prompt payment of expenses, large cash drawings and inadequate accounting records all make the task of book-keeping more difficult. Practice staff will naturally tend to gravitate to those employers who are organised and able to make their life easier.

ERROR 10   Have an affair!
Consultants do frequently, and inevitably, have a close working relationship with their secretarial and other support staff. Consultants are human beings and in some cases this relationship strays from being purely business. Staff affairs can have a disastrous effect on the efficiency and success of a practice. The old adage of 'business and pleasure do not mix' is particularly relevant in the small business structure of most consultant's practices.

The staff management errors listed above are commonplace. Most can easily be avoided. As indicated above, those consultants who are able to manage well, will reap the economic rewards. This is through a stable and dynamic staff structure, good patient relations and general economic efficiency.

4

Practice information and records

Successful businesses generally maintain a high standard of business records. This is to enable them to monitor and plan the business and to take corrective action as appropriate. Such a statement is so obvious it is perhaps remarkable that many consultants' practice records are of such poor quality. The need for quality records has been strengthened with the legal requirements following the introduction of the self assessment tax system. From 6 April 1996 it is now obligatory that all private practices maintain proper business books and records, and store them for at least seven years.

This chapter deals with some of the major business records required and the increasing role of computerisation. No attention is given to the precise nature of medical and patient records.

The basic books and records

The books that are required to be maintained by even the smallest medical practice are listed below. The precise format of the records, and whether they are computerised or not will depend on the nature and scale of the individual practice.

- *The fees ledger*: Consultants need to keep a record of all patient billing. Fee notes should at the very least include the date they were raised, details of the service provided and the cost to the patient. Insurance companies often request additional information, such as the procedure code. Fee notes should be numbered sequentially in order that records can be followed and checked. The fees ledger summarises the fees charged for each accounting period. For the smaller business, the fees ledger frequently acts as a debtors ledger, i.e. a record of what debts are outstanding. Typically a record is made of the date the fee note is actually paid. In this way, debtors outstanding at any moment of time can easily be identified.

- *The purchase ledger*: This ledger records details of invoices sent to the practice business from other suppliers. Typically, invoices relating to hospital fees, assistant fees, room hire and other related costs are sent to the practice. The purchase ledger records these invoices. For smaller practices, it is not uncommon for the purchase ledger to be used as a record of when payment has been made. In this way, the practice can immediately identify its debts to third parties.

- *The salaries/wages book*: As indicated in Chapter 3, there are now very strict rules on the operation of employees' remuneration through the PAYE system. The salaries book records payments made to staff and acts as a record for tax liability and payments under the PAYE system. Such records are particularly important as they may be required for audit by the Inland Revenue or the Department of Social Security.

- *The cash book*: This represents a record of cash payments into the practice from patients or insurance company receipts and cash payments out, for example to meet salaries, expenses or drawings. For many smaller practices, the bank account may suffice as the cash book, as long as it is independent from the consultant's private bank account.

- *The petty cash book*: Consultants are frequently very poor at recording small expenses which, in fact, are wholly legitimate as tax deductible expenses against their businesses. For example, tube fares, taxi fares, other travel costs, books, journals and refreshments are often not recorded. A simple petty cash book can act as a record for small items of expenditure. In addition, it can be used to record small items that are purchased for a consultant's office, such as stationery and postage.

- *The capital register*: Those in private practice are entitled to claim capital allowances against their taxable income for eligible capital expenditure. This may include, for example, medical equipment purchases, personal computers, office and consulting room fixtures and fittings, and their own motor vehicle. The capital register is a list of such fixed items that are purchased from time to time.

- *The travel diary*: With effect from 6 April 1998 tough new rules have been introduced governing the tax treatment of expenses for travel and subsistence. These rules will affect most consultants and medical practitioners who undertake private practice at different locations, NHS work at different sites or who act as a locum. Under the new rules, to obtain tax relief for travel from 6 April 1998, any journey must be made because it is a *requirement* or *obligation* of the job, rather than because a consultant or medical practitioner chooses to make it. Precise information is now needed on the precise nature of journeys and travel costs for both the consultant and his or her staff who travel regularly. Some specialist computer-based packages have recently come on to the market to assist in this respect.

To support these seven sets of basic records, it is essential that a practice business maintains copies of fee notes sent, invoices received and receipts for expenses claimed in order that documents can be checked or, if appropriate, records matched.

Suffice it to say that this daunting list of records is, in fact, much simpler to maintain in practice than in theory if adequate accounting systems have been installed.

The business bank account

Of all the records required by an efficient medical practice, the business bank account is perhaps the most important. A minority of consultants in practice do not maintain a business bank account.

They therefore lack the first line of any defence in the event of an investigation.

The advantages of a business bank account for a medical practice are several:

- first, it is a formal means of separating 'business' and 'private' matters. This automatically allows for better and easier monitoring of the financial performance and health of the practice

- second, it is a discrete record of transactions within the practice. A business bank account can easily be shown to any investigating Revenue officer without the need to explain, sometimes defensively, what is business and what is private

- third, the business bank account can become a useful financial planning tool. For example, fixed sums can be transferred as drawings to the private bank account where monies can be spent according to personal whim or need. Sums can be transferred by standing order to a tax deposit account, thereby acting as a savings device and reducing the need to worry about the need to find instant cash to meet tax demands

- fourth, the business bank account may reduce a consultant's overall bank charges. Any borrowings on a business account can be formalised and will generally attract an interest rate cost of base rate plus between 2 and 4%. Interest will be allowable against a consultant's tax bill if it is incurred wholly, necessarily and exclusively for the purpose of his or her business. Private bank accounts, if overdrawn without consent, can attract interest charges of up to 30% as well as daily unauthorised borrowing charges and heavy transaction fees. Interest is not tax deductible. In addition, interest on consultant's overdrawn private bank accounts is generally not allowed against tax, even if the account is used partially for business purposes

- fifth, the business bank account can make it easier to borrow efficiently and cost effectively. The bank manager can monitor the performance of a consultant's business through the bank account and can gain confidence in overall performance, without the impediment of having private and business affairs muddled.

Consultants express that there are some drawbacks in using business bank accounts. But to my mind these are minor relative to the overall advantages. Nonetheless, it is often stated that practice banking costs can increase as many banks offer 'nil cost' banking on private accounts, business bank accounts do not attract interest, and there is additional accounting and book-keeping work. Other consultants have stated that they do not wish to open a business bank account for fear of being subject to a barrage of pension, life assurance and other finance products now being marketed by the majority of bank managers. In my view this is no valid reason. Many consultants are, by their very nature, a key target for financial advisors and salesmen of whatever persuasion.

Computerisation of records

Computers are expanding rapidly into all areas of healthcare. As the pace of technology changes in the computer industry is accelerating rather than slowing down, the medical applications of new technology continue to increase. The whole medical sector has become a market growth opportunity for computer software companies to develop. Of particular relevance to private practices is the fact that all medical insurance companies are highly computerised and increasingly expect their suppliers to follow suit.

Computerisation is an absolute must for all forward-looking private medical practices. Tailor-made products have been on the market for some time. These include not only the basic accounting records described above, but also facilities for controlling the patient diary, patient records and the general practice management.

Many consultants still have an uneasy relationship with their computer. A number of common errors are made from the first decision to computerise the practice. If these are avoided the business will purchase and use computer systems appropriate to its precise needs.

ERROR 1   Do not plan for a computer
Those consultant businesses that purchase computers without planning their information requirements generally become

dissatisfied. Careful planning and specification in advance can assist a supplier to fully meet business needs.

ERROR 2   Select software by price alone
Many medical practitioners purchase software for their private practice based on price alone, perhaps not believing in the truth of the old adage that 'if you pay peanuts you get monkeys'. In reality, software should be selected on its ability to carry out predetermined tasks. Judgement must be made on suitability rather than affordability.

ERROR 3   Believe the marketing literature
Typically, consultants choosing computer systems will request marketing literature from a number of firms. Frequently marketing literature is designed to appeal to a predetermined target market, specifying key features and aiming to maximise sales. The standard software license agreement of most suppliers usually includes a clause to the effect that the supplier gives no warranty as to the suitability or otherwise of their software. The clear message is that of 'buyer beware'. The responsibility for selection falls on the consultant purchasers, who should request demonstrations and references from existing users.

ERROR 4   Forget to train staff
Staff training is essential to get maximum benefit from computer systems. Most software companies offer a specified number of hours training when they sell software. Prior to purchase, it is essential to clarify exactly what training is on offer. The more reputable suppliers will offer structured formal classroom training using test data. In other cases, the individual installing the software will use any spare time to quickly run through details. For most consultant businesses this training is of no use at all.

ERROR 5   Refuse to take up software support contracts and helpline
All reputable software houses offer a free telephone and software support, which is generally available during office hours to all new subscribers. Subsequently this may be offered on a fee-paying basis. Most consultant businesses generally require help in the first few weeks after installation. However, not uncommonly problems

arise after a year of use including, for example, the availability of memory as the volume of data increases, year end procedures where accounting information is held on the system and reporting procedures where data spans more than one year. With no software support contract a consultant is at the complete mercy of his or her computer system.

ERROR 6   Do not update the system regularly
For most consultants, computer hardware purchased is effectively obsolete the moment it is installed. Constant updating is necessary. Typically, problems arise when practices with computers decide to retain old hardware to run new software. In extreme cases there is a total lack of compatibility, resulting in additional software modification costs. More frequently, the new software may run more slowly on old equipment than old software. Regular updating of compatible hardware and software equipment is essential to avoid additional unbudgeted costs or disruption.

ERROR 7   Do not 'back up' the system
Compared to current hardware and software costs, tape back up systems are now relatively inexpensive. Data loss can prove to be a very expensive cost to a practice. The better-managed practices formally back up their data systems on a daily basis using written procedures. In this way, they ensure that the maximum time loss as a result of system failure is limited to one day. In the better practices, all staff are familiar with back up routines.

ERROR 8   Try to computerise all paper-based data
It is now possible to purchase software for a consultant to undertake virtually any task from planning the business diary to travel planning on holiday. Some consultants feel bullied by aggressive computer salesmen to try to computerise all aspects of their business. This temptation needs to be resisted as, in certain cases, paper-based systems are just as effective in performing a task and contributing to the smooth running of the practice.

ERROR 9   Eat in the office
It is not uncommon to see secretaries in medical practices eating their lunch over their computers. This innocent pastime should be

positively discouraged. One of the most effective ways of destroy-ing computer data and rendering the company inoperable is to introduce liquid into the processor. Wherever possible, it is in the interests of the practice to provide facilities so that food and drink can be consumed away from the computer and, perhaps of equal importance, out of the gaze of visiting patients.

ERROR 10   Introduce 'viruses'
Almost all large corporations now officially ban unsolicited computer software from being installed on their computer hard disks, smaller businesses are often not as rigorous. As a result of the large number of unlicensed computer disks available, it is possible to unwittingly introduce a computer 'virus' to the system. Viruses are frequently introduced through unlicensed computer game packages, which are loaded on to the computer by the medical secretary or operator. Viruses manifest themselves in different ways from reducing memory to actually deleting data.

Unquestionably computers and computerisation will play an ever-increasing role in private medical practice. Given the common errors listed above that are taken from actual consultants' experi-ence, it is essential to take the best advice available with regard to computers and computer software.

The problem of 2000 compliance

The much debated issue of the 'Year 2000 bug' concerns the treat-ment of the change of century by computer-based equipment and software which were developed without considering the implica-tions of the change in century numbers. The major problem is for systems that carry a two-digit field. These will commence the Year 2000 as 01/01/00 which in turn may treat the year as 1900.

While the potential problems have probably been exaggerated in the press, there is potential for disruption in private medical prac-tice businesses. The most common potential problems will relate to:

• any age-based calculations

• patient appointment recall systems where dates are a key factor

- staff salary, wages and sick pay systems

- aged creditor and debtors lists

- computer-based patient appointments and back-up schedules

- management reporting systems.

In addition to computers, consultants may face disruption in the performance of other equipment. This disruption includes, for example, consulting room alarms, fax machines, office heating and lighting controls, telephone machinery, any programmable machinery and any utility metering equipment. A three stage process can identify and possibly eliminate any dangers.

STAGE 1   Audit all equipment
All hardware and software equipment used in the medical practice should be listed in respect of its nature, its user, the location, its age and whether it is known to be '2000 compliant'. In addition, for equipment not compliant, a view needs to be taken of potential disruption ability. Target dates should be agreed for equipment needing to be tested.

STAGE 2   Test all equipment
Each item of equipment should be tested. In some cases, this may simply be confirmation from a supplier that it is '2000 compliant'. In other cases, professional assistance may be required.

STAGE 3   Check suppliers
Perhaps one of the greatest risks facing a medical consultant in private practice is that one of his or her suppliers' systems fails. The audit process, for completeness needs to be extended to suppliers as follows:

- Category 1 suppliers: these are generally corporate service providers, such as banks, insurance companies and utilities. Such suppliers will already, generally, have devoted considerable resources to ensure 2000 compliance

- Category 2 suppliers: these are generally medical service or equipment providers that are necessary for the consultant to perform his or her duties

- Category 3 suppliers: these are other suppliers to the business including, for example, business service and office goods.

As part of the audit process, a consultant should write to suppliers (particularly in category 2) requesting confirmation of compliance. Responses should be sought in writing and a simple 'register of compliance' kept. Those suppliers who are reluctant to cooperate or who have confirmed non-compliance should be viewed with suspicion.

Use of records in business control

Individual medical practices have different information require-ments. It is therefore difficult, if not impossible, to generalise. All medical practice businesses, however, are required to maintain records for income tax purposes, and the importance of accuracy and completeness in this respect has been fully emphasised above.

Records are also needed to control and plan the business. Used dynamically they can assist in improving performance and in providing guidelines to changes in policy and actions. In particular:

- to monitor the overall performance and productivity of the practice

- to monitor the cash requirement

- to enable the business to forecast and plan, for example in relationship to capital expenditure and taxation

- to enable the business to plan to meet creditor payments

- to enable the business to collect debts.

These matters are considered further in Chapter 11.

The principles of debt collecting

One of the most common problems facing medical practices is the collection of debts. This is no different from the problems facing any other professional-based practice. The quality of debt collecting varies considerably from consultant to consultant. However, a number of basic rules followed by the best practices appears to reduce the average number of debtor days outstanding and collection problems.

RULE 1   Raise clear fee notes
In general, fee notes should be precise and factual. Typically they should include the date, the patient name and address, the date of consultation(s) or of medical procedures, the dates of admission to hospital (if appropriate), details of the surgical or investigative procedure with the Office of Population Census and Statistics code (if appropriate) and the fee.

RULE 2   Check the fee note
It is remarkable how frequently consultants fail to send out an accurate fee note. Patient names and addresses are often wrong, dates misapplied and fees incorrectly computed. Errors in preparing fee notes will inextricably lead to delays in settlement.

RULE 3   Ensure that patients understand the method of charging and the basis of the fee
The best practices issue patients with what is effectively a fee tariff in advance of any consultation. This shows clearly the basis of charging and can be referred to in the event of any dispute. This process is particularly important if the consultant charges his or her fees at a different rate to that typically reimbursed to patients by leading insurance companies.

RULE 4   For insured patients seek direct settlement
Most insurance companies have now rectified the early technical problems they faced when introducing direct settlement schemes to consultants. Direct settlement reduces the problems frequently faced by consultants when their patients have received reimbursement from their insurance company, but they have not themselves yet issued a further cheque. In dealing with insurance companies, it is clearly essential to ensure that patient insurance details are fully understood by the practice administrators and that rules 1 and 2 are followed to the letter.

RULE 5   Offer a range of payment methods
Those consultants who have introduced credit or charge card machines and direct bank payment schemes have frequently been surprised at their success. Britain is increasingly a credit card society and there is a strong culture of acceptability of these cards as an immediate means of payment.

RULE 6   When in doubt – cash up front
Many consultants have not been reimbursed when they have given uninsured patients the benefit of the doubt. Consultants are in business to provide their services and there is no obligation for them to work in private practice without a guarantee of being paid. Payment before treatment can reduce future payment problems.

RULE 7   Introduce a strict credit control policy
On the assumption that a patient is aware of the practice credit terms, the practice secretary or administrator needs to rigidly enforce the policy. Typically, a credit control letter should be sent after 30 days, a follow-up telephone call after 45 days and a final 'letter before action' after 60 days. Longer-term delays typically reduce the prospect of being late. A consultant's value to his patients dissipates with time.

Prompt legal action to recover debts should follow after a 60-day period for maximum chances of recovery. Clearly there are exceptions to these rules, which a sympathetic consultant will take into account. However, a rigorously applied credit policy is essential for the smooth running of an efficient practice.

5

Practice pricing and marketing

The background to pricing of consultant's services

One of the major problems facing all medical consultants in practice is how to price his or her services to patients. The theory of pricing, as put forward by economists, is that prices charged are such that the demand for a service will equate to the supply of that service. With a fixed supply of gynaecology consultants, for example, a higher demand from patients will lead to higher prices. The 'market' will in turn respond to this situation by encouraging more gynaecology consultants into practice, with the result that prices to patients will fall as competition between clinicians increases. As new procedures become available demand from patients may increase, with the result that prices will rise again.

The theory is perfect, but practice in the medical sector is not. Historically, many consultants have opted to follow the BMA guidelines, and those of major insurance companies, such as BUPA. This comparatively simple situation changed with the advent of the Monopolies and Mergers Commission Report into the pricing of consultants' services in 1992. The Commission reported, perhaps with the benefit of current hindsight, that the BMA guidelines were contrary to the public interest in that they were tantamount to market price fixing. As a result, the BMA guidelines were outlawed. Paradoxically, BUPA price guidelines were not deemed to be against the public interest and, for many consultants, these have become the 'norm'.

The current situation is, that to all intents and purposes, BUPA guideline prices now predominate in the market. This is perhaps a rather surprising and unexpected result of the Monopolies and Mergers Commission report. BUPA and other insurance companies do not have the same interest in the efficiency of the market as the BMA and have academic economists. They are naturally interested in their own members and their profits and as such have a responsibility for reducing costs. Consultants and hospital fees are an obvious first target and in recent years insurance companies have followed a strategy of reducing these in real terms, with considerable success. While insurance companies have not yet gone so far as to introduce a formal 'black list' of consultants who they believe to be charging excessively high fees, they have managed to stem fee inflation through a variety of means. These include: a policy of unbundling of procedures; refusing to pay some consultants' fees; slow payment of consultants' fees; and the development of approved lists and so-called partnership agreements.

Many consultants in private practice have decided to follow a 'quiet life' policy and have acquiesced under the implicit and explicit pressure and influence of the insurance companies. The reality is, however, that consultants can determine the prices they charge patients. The obligations of insurance companies is to refund these charges to a certain and clear pre-stated level. There may be a difference that patients are prepared to fund if they are offered a significantly higher quality and standard of service.

Determination of fee rates

For those consultants who wish to determine their fee level there is little help available, apart from the published BUPA prices. There are, however, consultants who are able to fix and achieve fee levels which differ from these rates.

The key to determining an appropriate fee level is good information. This is needed both to establish initial fees for a new consultant and to adjust fee levels in a more mature business. An individual consultant, before publishing his or her fee rates, needs to gather a great deal of information both formally and informally. Much of this information is already available in the market. The following questions are typically asked:

- what are the BUPA published rates? Do these reflect the industry 'norm'?

- what are colleagues charging for similar work? It is always helpful, if possible, to gain copies of colleagues' tariffs. This is despite the fact that many consultants are tight-lipped when the question of fees is discussed

- what are the characteristics of the local marketplace in which the consultant operates? For example, fee rates can be influenced by the potential number of patients in the area, the distances they are prepared to travel, the age and socioeconomic structures of the local market; and the income structure of the potential patient market

- what is the nature of the competition?

- what is the consultant's episode cost of a particular treatment?

- is the consultant's episode cost greater or less than that achieved by the competition?

Experience has shown that the more complete the information base a consultant has on the nature of his or her market, his or her own skills and those of the competitors, the greater the ability to determine or maintain prices.

Once a consultant has assessed *external* market information, he or she needs to consider what he or she is offering to the market that is *unique* or *special*. For example:

- is the consultant offering total personal availability to patients, or is availability restricted?

- what is the average waiting time for a patient (for an initial appointment and in consulting rooms)?

- if the patient did not come to see the consultant, would he or she be prepared to visit the patient?
- what is the standard cost of a particular treatment, i.e. what charges would a patient incur if he or she went elsewhere?
- what does the consultant offer that is special? For example, does he or she offer a fast service, a low episode cost or a high first-time success rate?

In considering optimum fee levels, a consultant particularly needs to focus on what is special about his or her service in relation to the market and the competition. Consultants who can identify these factors can and do achieve premiums. Patients themselves are prepared to pay for unique or special care and service. The converse is also true. If a consultant can offer nothing special, services may have to be offered at a discount.

It is perhaps indicative of the way in which many consultants perceive themselves as naive businessmen or women that they underestimate their own abilities and skills, and the market's availability and willingness to pay for them. Careful and systematic examination of what they can offer their patients, combined with a thorough understanding of the marketplace, can lead to a pricing of their services which can maximise income through increasing overall fee levels.

Using fee levels to increase incomes

As indicated above, the first essential to formulating fee levels is to obtain information. Many consultants do rely on 'hearsay' and fix their prices on the basis of, in the economists' jargon, 'imperfect knowledge'. Given some knowledge, progressive medical practices can use pricing as a tool to boost income. Typical examples of alternative pricing methods include the following.

Determine pricing policies based on local income

Economists can demonstrate that one of the factors affecting the price of goods and services is income. Generally, the higher the level of income, the higher the price. Consultants can and should be able to charge higher prices for their services when they are working in higher-income areas than when they are working in lower-income areas.

Discount pricing at 'off-peak' times

Many public transport operators, for example, offer substantial discounts for off-peak travel. An increasing number of public houses and bars use the concept of 'happy hours' to attract business at off-peak times. Many consultants do have 'quiet' and 'busy' times of the week. Consultations and procedures could be offered at lower prices at off-peak times, and possibly at higher prices at antisocial times.

Premium pricing

The corollary of off-peak discount in the travel industry is premium pricing. Transport companies, for example, charge patients more at peak and busy times of the day. Many patients who want to take advantage of such times are often prepared, and able, to pay a premium.

Patient discounts/premiums

Travel companies frequently offer discounts to young passengers with limited income and elderly passengers with fixed incomes. Many consultants in practice currently charge the same price for a consultation to patients whatever their income or social structure. A more careful examination of a practice patient mix and introduction of appropriate discounts and premiums can attract more business and result in an income boost.

Let patients know prices

Economists have long argued that the more information there is available in any market, the more likely it is that there will be a genuine equilibrium price matching up supply and demand. British consultants are still generally very secretive about their consultation and procedure fees. Those consultants who do provide full and detailed information on their fee levels, often in the form of a restaurant type tariff, can frequently attract more patients.

Consider 'special deals'

Newspapers are full of 'special deals' in all areas of the economy. For example, supermarkets and airlines regularly offer 'special deals'. A consultant thinking imaginatively can often boost his or her income. For example, he or she may offer reduced prices for consultations and procedures in exchange for long-term patient commitment, or may consider 'special prices' at times of low demand for medical services in the calendar year or promotional arrangements when introducing new procedures or forms of consultation to the marketplace.

Package pricing

Perhaps the greatest opportunity of using pricing as a means to increase private practice incomes is through the technique of 'package pricing'. This technique has shown substantial growth in the economy in recent years. Weekend holiday breaks, overseas holidays, wedding arrangements and conferences are all good examples of where the consumer is looking to pay one price for a mass of goods and services.

The economist would argue that the advantages of package pricing are various:

- prices can be varied according to market conditions and constraints, for example, weather, time of year and time of day

- goods and services can be linked together to increase the income for a supplier

- sophisticated marginal pricing techniques can be used to increase margins and ultimately profits

- a stronger marketing message can be given to a consumer patient. Market research has shown that increasingly consumers are reluctant to accept 'extras' on their bills

- consumers are able to improve their budgeting. They can be clear, with good information, as to exactly what they are purchasing and how much it is costing.

The majority of the medical profession has still not adapted to the techniques of package pricing with any great enthusiasm. Often, following a consultation, a patient will be sent elsewhere for tests and will then have to return to the consultant for an interpretation. If he or she requires surgery there will be hospital fees, anaes-thetist's fees, surgeon's fees and often 'extras' to pay. A final consultation or even counselling may also be required. As a result, a number of suppliers of medical services will be raising fee notes or invoices to the patient or directly to the insurance company. The disadvantage of this system is that patients are often not aware in advance of the total cost of a treatment package. They are not therefore able to budget; they become resistant to a series of independent bills and as a result of the complex wording of many of their insurance company policies are not even sure as to the total extent of their medical cover.

A number of the more progressive medical consultants is now introducing package pricing to overcome these problems and is implicitly, taking advantage of the associated benefits. Those include increased patient flow, greater margins and, ultimately, higher incomes.

The trend towards 'package pricing' is accelerating. Consultants in private practice should consider carefully the relevance of this technique to their practices by pursuing a number of review steps relevant to their own particular business.

STEP 1   Identify the package
Most consultants are able to determine a standard range of packages which they, and their colleagues, offer to patients.

STEP 2   Identify the present constituent cost of the package
Most surgeons will be aware, for example, of the costs charged by their anaesthetists and by hospitals for standard ranges of services.

STEP 3   Identify how patients are currently billed
This procedure involves undertaking some informal market

research to establish what patients like and, of more importance, what they do not like.

STEP 4   Identify constraints and opportunities
There are times in the year, or in the week, when goods and services can be purchased more cheaply. For example, hospitals may be prepared to work for lower rates at 'off-peak' times. Conversely, there are times when there are constraints on the system and premiums to pay. The logic of such a review, for a consultant, is no different to that undertaken by package holiday planners.

STEP 5   Negotiate with suppliers
Once constraints and opportunities are identified, the consultant can negotiate with various suppliers of medical goods and services for their provision over a specific period. This can assist in planning. The golden rule in business in the late 1990s is that everything is negotiable!

STEP 6   Prepare pricing models
Based on the five-step analysis above, it is possible for consultants and their advisors to prepare alternative pricing models for standard goods and services. For example, in the case of breast surgery, this may mean offering a package price to patients covering all consultations, hospitalisation, surgeon's fees, anaesthetist's fees and postoperative counselling.

STEP 7   Market effectively
Once a service package has been determined, and costs agreed, marketing literature can be prepared. The objective of this literature is to give prospective patients a clear view of what is on offer for the package price. Professional marketing assistance may be necessary to ensure that a fully professional package, consistent with medical ethics guidelines, is prepared.

Some consultants will doubtless find the infiltration of more specific and management accounting techniques and the influence of marketing in their practices to be anathema. However, in my view, if they do not introduce these techniques or if they fail to become more sophisticated in pricing and marketing, they will fall behind others in their income earning ability. The example of the holiday industry is clear. There are still independent, intrepid travellers and some totally independent hotels. However, the tourist industry is now completely dominated by the concept of 'packages' at both the most extravagant and humble ends of the market.

Marketing the practice: the need to act professionally

There is still a strangely ambivalent attitude towards marketing from the medical industry's professional body, the GMC. For many years, the GMC held the view that any advertising or marketing of professional services by consultants was unbecoming of the dignity of the profession. Following substantial market changes in the 1980s and 1990s, the restriction of rules and the opening up of professional marketing for other professionals, notably accountants and solicitors, and specific pressure from the Monopolies and Mergers Commission, the GMC has amended its views.

The GMC changed its guidelines for advertising and marketing in 1990. The principal effects of these changes were that:

- advertising through the provision of factual information became possible

- information provided must in no circumstance denigrate, or be seen to denigrate, the quality and skills of other professional medical services

- material issued by doctors must comply with the British code of advertising and must be 'legal, decent, honest and truthful'

- any advertising or other material issued must not put patients at risk or mislead them in any way.

The changes introduced in 1990 seemed to give far greater marketing opportunities to GPs than to consultants. While the GMC stated that, after 1990, it had 'no objection' to specialists providing information to GPs and other professional colleagues, it did prohibit providing information directly to the public, except in limited circumstances. The rationale for this view was that it was designed to protect individual patients who may be sufficiently ill or susceptible to published material made available by the consultant. In my view, this logic is weak and market events have shown that some consultants have extended what may be regarded as legitimate commercial marketing activity.

Nonetheless, given the apparent initial grudging acceptance by the GMC of the role of the marketplace, it is important that any specialist ensures he or she operates within current ethical guidelines and codes of conduct set down and interpreted at the time. Professional advice from the GMC and possible clearance is essential on areas of marketing and promotion which appear to be commercially acceptable but professionally contrary to guidelines. Anything that is written below must be interpreted in this context.

Marketing the practice: the network

In most professional businesses there are three types of individuals: the 'finder', the 'minder', and the 'grinder'. The 'finder' finds and negotiates the business; he or she markets and sells the business service. The 'minder' supervises the work. And the 'grinder' does the work. An individual consultant in private practice encompasses all three roles.

One of the key roles of the 'finder' is to utilise, as far as possible, market research. I have indicated above that detailed market research is an essential prerequisite for the determination of individual and package pricing. The key element of market research in establishing, developing and holding together a private practice is the so called 'network'. This is effectively the means by which patient flow is generated and held. Specifically for a consultant developing a practice it is important to understand, both statically and dynamically, the 'network'. This comprises:

• the key GP referrers of patients of relevance to him or her. Names may be available, for example from NHS statistics

- the key GP non-referrers of patients. Through this information, marketing campaigns can be focused. As a guideline, for many successful consultants, 80% of the patient flow will originate from 20% of their GP referrers

- the key professional players in the local market, e.g. the principal competitor consultants and, for surgeons, the key anaesthetists

- other key players of importance in the marketplace. For example, these may include administrators or nursing staff who have a significant influence on patient flow.

The network database is a significant asset to the successful practice. The more progressive consultant business will have this computerised and regularly updated and reviewed.

Marketing the practice: the tools

A range of tools is available for any private medical consultant marketing his or her services. These are listed below. It should be noted that the first eight tools listed raise no ethical questions whatsoever.

1. *The skills of the consultant*: The professional skills and reputation of the consultant are critical to formulation of ongoing marketing campaigns. Reputations are enhanced and destroyed by word of mouth. Paradoxically, it takes far less time to destroy a reputation than it does to create one. Constant attention to maintenance and toning of professional skills is therefore essential, both in the NHS and in private practice. In this respect, academic papers may help to create an image of skill and professionalism. However, for the successful consultant it is the day-in, day-out quality of his or her performance in both the NHS and his or her private practice that are most important.

2. *The personality of the consultant*: Highly skilled consultants can have poor private practices. The converse is true. The more successful consultants in private practice tend to be those who are personable, friendly and popular. Aggressive or sub-

missive consultant personalities do not help in the marketing of their business.

3. *The availability of the consultants*: The market increasingly demands constant availability from its medical professionals. Those consultants who make themselves available, despite possible personal inconvenience, have a strong marketing tool. Those who establish strong time constraints and are generally unavailable have discarded the use of a strong marketing tool. A straw poll suggests that those consultants engaged heavily in, for example, NHS or industry politics generally have a weaker private practice than those who do not.

4. *Presentability of the consultant*: For the majority of patients and their referrers, a tidy, well-dressed, presentable consultant is a marketing plus. Poorly dressed, shabby consultants who may excel technically give a market impression of slovenliness.

5. *Ambience of the consulting rooms*: Light, tidy neat rooms are a very positive marketing tool. Untidy, poorly decorated rooms with worn furniture discourage referrers and patients.

6. *Professionalism of support staff*: Well-dressed, polite, trained and competent support staff enhance a practice image. Incompetent, impolite and badly dressed or postured staff inhibit its growth. A surprising number of private medical practices have not developed directly as a result of the incompetence and image of the practice secretary and the reluctance of the proprietor to do anything about it.

7. *Traditional advertising*: These techniques consist of the telephone directory entry, the door plate and the standard letter new consultants often send to GPs. While these are appropriate marketing tools, in my view they are relatively minor in their impact.

8. *Pricing*: Considerable attention has been given above to the theory and practice of pricing. For many businesses, pricing flexibility and originality offer a significant marketing tool.

9. *'Patient packs'*: Increasingly, consultants in successful private practices prepare 'patient packs'. These comprise factual

details of services offered, details of what happens to patients undergoing treatment, names and addresses of appropriate sources of information and a tariff of prices. While these are now primarily handed to referred patients, they can be used as advertising material, with copies given to referrers.

10. *Formal meetings*: Perhaps the most common marketing tool is the formal meeting between a consultant in his capacity as a 'finder' and a GP referrer of patients. Experience suggests that such meetings are more effective at a GP's rooms, where there is a small number present and where there is follow up. A well-prepared and presented case of the consultant services and special skills is essential to the formal meeting.

11. *Informal meetings*: Inevitably, some consultants adopt the 'informal meeting' tool as part of their ongoing marketing programme. For example, this may include provision of dinners or invitations to sports events. This technique is quite common in most areas of business and can be used to increase the level of bonding, particularly where an initial professional relationship has been established.

12. *Other tools*: There is a range of other marketing tools whose worth is often difficult to determine. These may include, for example, newspaper and journal advertisements, articles and advertorials, and radio and television appearances. In certain instances these may be of particular benefit to practices. However, the science of marketing techniques has far exceeded the ability of current thinking on ethical advertising and advice from the GMC is probably essential if some or all of these techniques are considered.

Marketing strategy

For all private medical practices marketing is an ongoing function. Sadly, many consultants do not devote the time, energy and persistence that is necessary for successful marketing. Some underestimate their worth and ability as marketers, while others find the whole process demeaning and unprofessional. However, the reality is that those practices that are marketed well are generally the most successful financially.

Individual marketing campaigns are more successful if they are tailored to the specific private medical practice. Any guidelines to specific strategy can therefore be no more than a series of tips.

TIP 1   Regularly monitor the success of marketing
In this respect, formal and systematic review of the sources of new patients is the simplest technique.

TIP 2   Regularly review the efficiency of marketing tools listed as (1)–(9) above
These are often considered to be standard marketing tools which are the 'norm' in any professional private practice. Any weaknesses do need to be considered and acted upon instantly.

TIP 3   Maintain a regular pattern of meetings
The referral network is, for most private medical practices, the key means by which business is generated and maintained. Establishment of a regular time commitment to meetings (both formal and informal) with GPs and others is a key element to an effective marketing strategy. Suffice it to say, it is incumbent upon the consultant to have something to say at a meeting, and detailed preparation is essential. For example, episode costings, speed of service, follow up rates and new services offered are all standard themes around which meetings can be structured.

TIP 4   Take professional advice on literature
Poorly designed and prepared literature of any kind is a marketing disadvantage. The professional preparation of all literature (including letterheads, 'with compliments' slips, invoices and patient packs) frequently generates significant rewards.

TIP 5   Constantly review and be very clear on what services are on offer
Consultants in private practice frequently do not have a clear objective of what they are selling and their unique selling proposition (i.e. what it is they have that is special). Some spread their efforts and allow themselves to become distracted. Such a diffu-

sion of effort reduces the efficiency of any marketing efforts. The well versed, but simple piece of American advice is true: 'Stick to the Knitting'!

TIP 6   Be persistent

Marketing, for a sole consultant in private practice, can frequently be a lonely and seemingly unrewarding activity. For those times when marketing effort seems to be unrewarding, the so-called 'Cook guiding principles' may give some comfort:

Press on.

Nothing in the world can take the place of persistence.

Talent will not; nothing is more common than unsuccessful men with talent; genius will not; unrewarded genius is almost a proverb.

Education will not; the world is full of educated derelicts.

Persistence and determination alone are omnipotent.

(Andrew Cook, Chairman's Statement,
William Cook Cast Products)

6

Finance and banking

Source of finances

The clearing bank is the most obvious and frequently used source of finance for a new consultant practice, and for one expanding. A whole range of financial products is, in theory, available to the consultant or his or her advisor who has researched the market. The principal products utilised by consultants in private practice are:

- the short-term overdraft, typically used to finance working capital and to fund timing differences in the business cycle

- medium-term loan, typically used to finance capital purchases or the hard-core element of an overdraft and negotiated between a one- and 15-year period

- the long-term loan, typically negotiated to acquire a practice premises, and negotiated for up to 20 years

- leasing, which can take two principal forms, lease purchase and contract hire. Lease purchase finance agreements provide consultant businesses with the use and eventual ownership of new and used assets. Typically these agreements will run for between two and five years, at the end of which legal ownership of the assets is with the consultant. Under an operating lease contract and a contract hire arrangement, title to the assets will remain with the finance provider.

Other sources of finance, such as factoring, invoice discounting, loan facilities under the terms of the Small Firms Loan Guarantee Scheme and equity, are available in the market but at present are infrequently used by medical practices. Business circumstances change and unquestionably these forms of finance will become more commonplace in progressive practices.

The role of the bank in the development of private medical practice

Increasingly, commercial banks are looking towards what they regard as a 'partnership' with their medical customers. Their own research has told them that customers are looking for a more proactive approach including:

- innovative financial solutions that can be tailored to specific customer requirements

- excellent standards of service

- value for money

- understanding by the bank of their customers' business

- continuity of contact.

Bankers have identified that to enable them to assist their customers they do require an efficient exchange of information. For most consultants, this involves the supply of accurate annual practice accounts presented in a timely fashion. However, for practices that are expanding and looking for bank support for finance, banks are increasingly looking behind and around the figures. For instance, they are showing increasing interest in other areas of a consultants' business including the quality of management, the product and marketing strategies adopted, pricing policies and capital investment programmes.

It is impossible for a consultant to run his practice without using the services of a bank of some sort. To run his or her business well, there needs to be:

- a good relationship with the bank manager

- attention to detail in managing the relationship with the bank. This involves much more than simply understanding and sticking to the terms and conditions of any bank finance being provided. The handling of the relationship, from a consultant's viewpoint is critical to long-term growth.

Handling the bank

The more successful private practice businesses have learnt to handle their banks through a variety of means. These are summarised as follows:

- by ensuring that the bank understands the precise nature of the consultant's business, its needs and cycles

- by ensuring that the bank conducts its business with the consultant in accordance with its own code of practice. All banks now operate a code of practice. It is incumbent for consultants to obtain a copy of this code, and if the bank is deviating from its own written standards to advise it accordingly

- by accepting that 'knowledge is power'. A consultant should always know what his or her facilities are, how they work and what they cost. Small print of any documentation should be read and understood. With this knowledge, any changes or errors made by the bank (and they are increasingly made!) can be corrected and adjusted in the least possible time and at least expense

- by never being pressured into an agreement that does not seem right. Banks do have their own targets for performance, and they not infrequently offer consultant businesses, which are frequently financially naive, using products and terms that are not appropriate. They will also often pressure consultants to take up their own range of financial products, such as life assurance, key man assurance and pensions. The advice is always to resist terms that are not appropriate. The market is free and new banks are often pleased to take on quality business on different terms

- by never being wrong-footed. Consultant businesses should always seek to replace, negotiate and extend their financing arrangements in good time. With banks, timeliness is next to godliness!

- by ensuring that the lines of communication are maintained. In recent years, there have been major changes in bank personnel and these are likely to continue. Consultants often face the prospects of dealing with new and inexperienced managers. Under the current bank policies of 'partnership', insistence that the bank visits the practice consulting rooms is an appropriate means of ensuring continuity

- by recognising your own financial weaknesses. Problems will often arise with a consultant's banker if it fears that he or she is running into trouble and trying to hide the fact. The best advice is not to keep embarrassing secrets and not to spring surprises on the bank

- by taking the initiative when finance is required. A well thought through budget and, as appropriate, business plan is an essential aide to support a borrowing request. Best practice would advise that a borrowing request be supported by three projections – one covering the current outlook, one covering an improving scenario and one covering a deteriorating worst-option scenario. Taking the initiative also suggests maintaining constant financial vigilance, and advising the bank when there is a change of circumstances.

Ways to upset the bank manager

As indicated above, the relationship with the bank is probably the only significant financial one that most private medical practice businesses will have. It is therefore perhaps surprising that a number of consultants in practice, particularly those newly started, can frustrate this relationship to their businesses disadvantages. Common errors are listed below.

ERROR 1 Prepare accounts late
Historically, medical practitioners were considered a safe bet. Bank managers were almost laxadaisical in their timing of request

for practice accounts. Times have changed, and they are subject to the careful scrutiny of the computer and their own internal auditor. Prompt submission of practice accounts, whether simple or complex, establishes in the banker's mind a feeling of orderliness and efficiency. Late accounts lead bankers to think of inefficiency and lack of business acumen.

ERROR 2   Don't prepare accounts
An even worse sin, in the eyes of bank managers is not to prepare accounts at all. This is true, even for the smallest of practices.

ERROR 3   Ask for more finance than is needed
Bankers thrive on well thought out budgets and cash flows which indicate the quantum and timing of bank support required. Those who are prepared to support their borrowing requests with data, statistically stand more chance of success. Paradoxically those who request and receive a facility which is not used are penalised when it comes to a renewal. Bankers live by selling utilised facilities.

ERROR 4   Ask for less finance than is needed
Excess borrowing can be very expensive, in terms of high penalty interest rate charges and additional costs imposed on the borrower. In addition, bankers are normally very reluctant, in the first instance, to 'bounce' cheques. Once they have taken the step to bounce a practitioner's cheque for the first time, they will have far fewer inhibitions on a later occasion.

ERROR 5   Complain constantly
Sadly, improvements in banking technology have not reduced the propensity for error. There are increasing examples of overcharging, and all consultants are advised, as a precaution, to check costs imposed. When challenged, most banks will remedy errors. However, bankers are human and a constantly complaining consultant is unlikely to receive the best support. When the propensity to complain becomes high, the advice is for the consultant to change banks.

ERROR 6   Regularly change banks
All banks are in the business of attracting new customers.

Newspapers are full of special 'deals' and incentives for new customers. It is unnatural for consultants not to be tempted by these offers and to seek to transfer their bank regularly. Such constant moves do not allow a banker, or more realistically his competition, to build up a profile and trading record of his customer.

ERROR 7   Avoid professional help
A large number of medical practitioners still seeks to negotiate its own banking and overdraft arrangements. A little knowledge is frequently dangerous, and many practitioners find themselves being overcharged, paying uncompetitive interest rates, carrying bank-imposed life assurance and incurring heavy service charges. Professional help can identify the appropriate finance product required and its price.

ERROR 8   Live a noticeably good lifestyle in relation to income
Banking, as a profession, is no longer secure or well paid. Bankers do study their customers' living habits and know a surprising amount about them. Expensive private schools for children of newly established consultants, exotic holidays, fast cars and costly mistresses or lovers are all noticed. Bankers are increasingly reluctant to finance what they perceive to be a consultant's excessive life style. They have the power to terminate a lifestyle, through withdrawal of facilities at an instance.

ERROR 9   Don't pay the revenue
Banks are nervous when their medical clients do not meet tax bills on time. This is because the Revenue is a preferential creditor, and in cases of difficulty can take priority in payment terms over a bank.

ERROR 10   Ignore bank correspondence
As bankers themselves become more defensive as a profession, increasingly requests and comments are committed to writing. Unanswered or delayed responses to bank letters is generally a panacea for trouble.

Despite the apparent bank philosophy of resorting to 'partnership relationships' as described above, in my view, the relationship between a banker and his or her medical practitioners is becoming more ordered and regulated and therefore less personal. This is primarily the result of ongoing technological changes. Increasing discipline and attention to the banker's needs is paramount to the development of the relationship. Those consultants who do recognise the changing environment can rely on the support of the banker in developing their business. Those who ignore this, and regularly commit some or all of the 10 relationship errors listed above, can expect to pay a high price for their borrowings, if indeed they can negotiate any.

7

Taxation

Probably more time is spent on attempting to reduce taxation liability in private medical practices than in seeking to maximise post-tax income. This suggests that taxation minimisation is an extremely important business objective for a significant majority of medical practitioners.

The subject of taxation is complex and professional advice is essential on points of detail and where problems arise. Nonetheless there are matters of general principle that can impact on the operation and performance of private medical practices.

General principles

For the majority of consultants in private practice, whether trading as an individual or in a partnership of some kind, tax on earnings will be assessed as self-employed under Schedule D rather than under Schedule E, the schedule applicable to employed earners (e.g. salaried employees working in the NHS). For the minority trading as limited liability companies, taxation will be assessed under corporation tax rules. A summary of the significant tax rates as from 6 April 1998 is given in Appendix A.

While it is not the purpose of this book to act as a tax text, a number of significant observations apply.

- The tax regime under Schedule D and corporation tax rules is more liberal as regards the offset of expenses against income. Expenses that are 'wholly and exclusively' can be offset against income under the rules. For Schedule E income earners expenses will only be allowed if they are 'wholly, exclusively *and* necessarily' incurred in the performance of an employment. Schedule E expenses are ones that all medical practitioners are liable to incur and which are *essential* to that employment. In practice, the tough rules on Schedule E earnings often mean that professional subscriptions are often the only deductible expenses claimed and allowed.

- Claims can be made against income for so-called capital allowances. These are tax reliefs given against business capital expenditure (such as medical equipment and consulting room furniture) at predetermined rates. In addition, allowances can be made for use of private cars, though these are restricted. The current capital allowance rates are summarised in Appendix A.

- Taxable profits from private practice are normally assessed on an earnings basis, i.e. the fee notes invoiced during a financial year (not necessarily monies collected) with deductions for costs incurred (not actually paid). Some consultants' taxable profits are, however, assessed on a 'cash' basis (i.e. tax is paid on monies actually received less an allowance for expenses actually paid out). This method may have cash flow advantages in certain situations. However, in an Inland Revenue press statement dated 22 December 1997 it was stated that the 'cash' basis of preparing medical consultants' private practice accounts, along with that of other professionals, is being withdrawn. This will be replaced by the new accruals basis of accounting from tax year 1999–2000. Professional advice will be necessary at the time on the implications to a particular business of the changes. In time, 'cash' accounting for consultants will become an historical anachronism.

- The taxpayer is responsible for the assessment of tax. With the advent of self assessment the consultant is now legally responsible for the computation and payment of his or her tax liability. There are strict time limitations and target dates, which need to be adhered to. These are considered below. Under present arrangements, corporation tax has to be paid nine months after an accounting year end on the so-called 'pay and file' basis. This system is due to change from 1 July 1999 to bring companies into line with the individual and partnership self assessment rules.

- Full records have to be maintained of practice affairs and finances. These matters were considered in Chapter 4.

- The consultant trading as a sole trader or in partnership will be subject to Class 2 and Class 4 national insurance contributions. There are exemptions for those who have employment income, say from the NHS, in excess of £25 220 per annum, from 6 April 1998. However, proper exemption claims have to be made to the Department of Social Security, and it is surprising how many newly established consultants fail to deal adequately with registering for exemption of Class 2 and Class 4 national insurance contributions.

Allowable expenses

While the guide is not definitive, and each individual case needs to be considered on its merits, the following typical expenses are allowed against a practice income taxed under Schedule D.

Allowability	Expense items
(i) 100% relating to private practice business	Accounting, legal and other professional expenses; bad debts written off; claims for professional negligence (excess only not covered by insurance); conference expenses; consulting-room repair, maintenance, decoration and rental; hire purchases, bank and other interest paid (except cars); laundry and cleaning; medical journals and periodicals; medical supplies; travel expenses and reasonable

refreshments, excluding home to consulting room; printing, stationery and postage; professional subscriptions (though usually more efficient to claim against Schedule E); protective and special clothing; repairs and renewals; secretarial assistance, staff salaries and assistants' fees, consulting room, telephone, fax and Internet expenses; training expenses and costs, which require existing skills; waiting-room decoration, journals and flowers.

In addition, companies are allowed to make pension contributions for their consultant directors, on the understanding that they are supported by actuarial computations. Contributions are generally wholly allowable.

(ii) Proportion of expenses allowed

Costs of maintaining and running one or more private cars in so far as these relate to business use; costs of maintaining an element of private residence expenses used by the business (including heat and light, rates, repairs, insurance; proportion of interest paid on hire purchase or bank loans relating to business use of one or more vehicles); home telephone and fax calls relating to business use (rentals generally not allowable).

(iii) Expenses allowed according to capital allowance rules

• For plant, machinery and medical equipment, 25% on a reducing balance (40% of cost for the first year from 2 July 1998).

- For motor cars, 25% on a reducing balance with a maximum of £3000 pa. This is subject to deduction for private use.
- Scientific research, 100% allowable.
- Know how, 25% on reducing balance.
- Patent rights, 25% on reducing balance.

For many medical practitioners the principal difficulty has been with the proportion of business expenses claimed with respect to motor vehicle and use of private residence costs. Historically, the determination of the rate has been something of a horse trade with H M Inspector of Taxes, with the onus of benefit frequently lying with the consultant. Under the new self assessment rules, the onus of proof has changed. Much fuller information is required to support a claim, which can be challenged by the Revenue in any audit. As a guide:

- if the home, or a proportion of it, is used for business purposes (for example, as consulting rooms or a private office), the general rule is that a proportion of expenses can be claimed, commensurate to the total area of the home. Some allowance can be made for 'service' areas, such as bathroom and kitchen, if required for business use. Accurate measurement is essential, and it is important for the consultant to *actually use* the space at home for business purposes for which he or she is claiming

- if such claims are made, there may be a proportional capital gains tax liability if the home is sold. While there are undoubtedly cases, these are, in practice, extremely rare

- for motor vehicles, full recording of costs with receipts, is necessary. Consultants are often lax in collecting full cost receipts and, as a general rule, credit card vouchers are not good enough

- in addition to the full cost record, it is now advisable to maintain a full record of business journeys as proof of business use. The proportion of business use can then be assessed, subject to taking a view on how essential a motor vehicle is in the event of emergency requirements

- the additional records for self assessment will mean, in time, that probably supportable and documented claims for use of the home and business use of motor vehicles will reduce for many consultants. Implicitly, this is a gradual withdrawal of a Schedule D privilege.

Self assessment: the key dates

Much has been written on the self assessment system and consultants in practice will already have had at least a year's experience. One of the key features in managing this new system is the need to adhere to the key dates very precisely.

The initial essential date was 6 April 1996, the first date of the 'records' regime. Up to this date, a tax inspector had to have a reasonable suspicion that a consultant's tax affairs were not in order to institute an inspection or enquiry. From 6 April 1996, this constraint has been removed, and a consultant's affairs can be reviewed at any time, for no stated reason, by an inspector. From this date there is a statutory obligation to maintain records, and those consultants who are lacking in this respect will face fines and possible penalties.

The self assessment cycle is now driven by key dates in the financial year calendar. These dates need to be incorporated into the practice business calendar:

6 April   The Revenue will issue self assessment returns covering income for the previous year to 5 April.

19 May   The last date for consultants, in their capacity as employers, to submit PAYE year-end forms P35 for the previous year to 5 April. Many consultants forget to submit these returns, even though they may only be paying their wives (or husbands) a salary.

30 May   The last date by which employees of consultants'

business may receive their forms P60 for income to the previous 5 April.

6 July   The last date by which a consultant employer may submit to the Revenue forms P9D and P11D in respect of their employees who are paid expenses or receive any benefits in kind. Employees are entitled to receive copies of these forms.

31 July   The second date of payment of tax on account. For example, the second payment on account for the 1997/98 tax year was due on 31 July 1998.
In addition, if tax returns and computations for the previous year are still outstanding there will be a £100 penalty and a surcharge of 10% on tax unpaid. On 31 July 1998 these penalties will be applicable on all tax returns outstanding to 5 April 1997.

30 September   This is the last date for consultants to submit their tax returns on income to the previous 5 April *if they want the Revenue to calculate their tax liability*.
This is also the deadline for notifying the Revenue of any new sources of income.

5 October   The last date for notifying the Revenue of any chargeable gains for the previous financial year.

31 January   The last date for submission of tax returns for the year to the previous 5 April together with any self assessment of computation of liability and payment of tax due. The date is also the date of the first payment on account of the current year's tax, based on the liability for the previous year. For example, on 31 January 1999, the balance of tax due for 1997/98 will become payable as well as the first payment on account for 1998/99. Automatic fines of £100 are imposed if the returns are not received by this date.

28 February   The date of first surcharge of 5% of tax not paid. For example, a 5% surcharge will be imposed on any 1997/98 tax not paid by 28 February 1999.

In addition to the tax surcharges imposed on tax not paid on 28 February and 31 July each year, interest will be charged. As a further cost burden, interest will be charged on unpaid surcharges.

For many consultants in private practice the key date, in terms of financial planning is 31 January. This is the date for payment of the balance of the previous year's tax and payment on account of 50% of the estimated current year's tax. Those whose practices are growing rapidly will find particularly heavy tax bills due on this date. A sensible precaution is to set aside each month an estimated proportion of monies due in order that the tax bill can be met and embarrassment minimised.

Self assessment: consultants' experiences

Inevitably there have been teething problems arising from the introduction of a new tax system. The Inland Revenue has argued that over 90% of taxpayers submitted their returns by 31 January 1998, with a much lower error rate than expected. On the other hand, one of the leading accountancy bodies, the Chartered Association of Certified Accountants, has pointed to a trail of error, delay and miniscule tax demands.

A number of clear observations has arisen from dealing with consultants' affairs in the new tax regime.

- Consultants have generally met their tax requirements on time and have completed with the dates schedules identified above.

- Revenue processing of returns has often been slow and inaccurate. In cases where the Revenue has offered to calculate tax due, there appear to have been incorrect statements, late statements, threatening demands and a general slow-down in the speed at which correspondence has been dealt with. Where there have been Revenue errors, it is well worth complaining.

- The accuracy and completeness of many consultants' financial records and systems still leaves much to be desired. A significant number of consultants do not maintain accurate records of their mileage and travel expenses, their business operating costs or, in extreme cases, even their billing.

- Tax planning has become more difficult. The slow-down in Revenue response rates has meant that adjustments have not been implemented as speedily as previously. In addition, changes in the interpretation of rules has meant, for example, that some consultants paying personal pension contributions have had to pay tax demands in full, and subsequently make claims for tax relief on contributions. Tax-efficient pension planning is an important matter for those consultants and these changes have increased practical management problems.

- The computer has taken over. Over the past year or so, many consultants have received a significant number of pre-programed computer documents. In extreme cases, these documents have borne no relationship to previous documents and have caused stress and much additional work.

Tips to handle self assessment in future

Based on consultants' practical experiences, some seven tips have emerged to handle the self assessment system.

TIP 1   Deal with tax affairs promptly
Those consultants who have dealt with the tax affairs early in the financial year have generally had fewer Revenue problems. They have also been better able to plan their finances to meet tax demands.

TIP 2   Improve the quality of business records
This is a consistent theme of this text.

TIP 3   Notify any changes in personal or business circumstances early
Despite the slowdown in Revenue response rates, letters do remain on file, and can be used as evidence in the event of any future problems or investigations.

TIP 4   Where appropriate, chase employers and others for salary, benefits and information as required
As indicated above, such documents should be supplied not later than 6 July in any tax year.

TIP 5   Deal with computer-generated demands or statements promptly
Do not leave these documents unattended.

TIP 6   Try to submit returns by 30 September
This allows an opportunity for the Revenue to calculate tax, and for the more orderly processing of documents.

TIP 7   Have some sympathy with your accountant
Professional surveys in the accountancy profession have show that many have spent up to 33% more time on individual client affairs than in previous years. Consultants have been notably resistant to approve increasing accounting fees.

Tax investigations

From 31 January 1998, the Revenue operates under new rules relating to tax investigations of a consultant's affairs. Under these rules, the Revenue has power to institute:

- a 'full enquiry' into the books and records maintained by a consultant. This is similar in concept to an 'in-depth' investigation under the old rules

- an 'aspect' enquiry, whereby the Revenue can investigate a particular point in a tax return. Often such an enquiry will be of a highly technical nature.

From January 1998, there are four factors that can institute an enquiry into a medical practitioner's affairs:

1. A genuine random audit. The Revenue has stated it will be randomly auditing about 0.1% of tax returns received. On the assumption that there are about 17 500 practising consultants

and 30 000 registrars and other qualified doctors within the NHS, only about 50 or so per annum will have their affairs reviewed by the random audit process.

2. The 'level of income' analysis. The Revenue has classified all tax payers into six groups, viz. small business (with a turnover of less than £15 000), medium business (with a turnover of £15–£250 000), large business (with a turnover of £250 000 and over), very large business, non-business and others. A significant number of consultants with private practice income will be classified into the 'small' or 'medium' business group. These are the groups that the Revenue has stated will be heavily targeted for full enquiry work. In addition, the Revenue has stated that it will undertake automated risk assessments of returns. Those consultants who, for example, have unsatisfactory rates of gross profits, inexplicable income changes or low personal drawings will carry a higher risk of investigation. Such 'risk groups' will be held on a consultant's file, to assist the Revenue Compliance Manager in deciding whether or not to open an enquiry.

3. Mandatory review. Certain matters will in future be flagged up to a Revenue Compliance Manager to make a decision as to whether he or she institutes a full, an aspect or indeed no enquiry. Typical events will be:

   – where a medical practitioner has included provisional figures in his or her tax return

   – where a medical practitioner has failed to notify chargeability on any aspects of his or her income

   – where the Compliance Manager thinks for whatever reason, that a medical practitioner is adopting an unsatisfactory attitude to the self assessment system generally.

4. 'Shopping'. The concept of 'shopping' is increasing in the medical sector. For example, consultants may be reported to the Revenue anonymously if they are undertaking private work that is in any way inconsistent with the terms of their NHS contract.

In addition to the inherent 'high risk' problems of private medical practice as an entity liable to investigation, particular aspects of a practice may attract an inspector's attention. Common features include:

- where there is a high proportion of foreign patients in the practice, with a propensity for cash transactions
- where there is plenty of 'sub-contract' labour utilised, for example, through paying of assistant's fees
- where there are high claims for use of home. Inspectors have been known to visit consultant's homes to verify the accuracy of claims
- where consultants seek to prepare their own accounts and do not utilise professional assistance
- where the consultant's appointments book is regularly thrown away at the end of each year
- where the consultant maintains an extrovert lifestyle
- where salaries to wives and/or husbands for working in the practice are high
- where consultants have plenty of cash in their wallets and in their safe at home.

It would seem logical that, given the four means by which a tax enquiry may now start, the chances of a typical consultant in practice being the target of the Revenue's attentions has increased.

The institution of an enquiry

There is a fixed procedure by which the Revenue can institute an enquiry. It now has to institute a formal 'notice of intended investigation', and there are rigorous rules that apply, designed to protect both the Revenue and the taxpayer. On completion of an enquiry, a formal 'completion notice' now has to be issued. As a general rule, professional help should be sought once a consultant, or an immediate member of his or her family, receives a 'notice of intended investigation'.

The 'lifestyle' test

The means by which the Revenue can investigate a consultant's affairs are various. One of the most common methods, and potentially disruptive, is the so-called lifestyle test. This is often applied where the Revenue believes that a consultant has, for whatever reason, understated his or her income and/or overstated expenses that have been claimed.

In essence, the object of the test is to compare an individual's, or often a family's, net cash receipts in a year with their expenditure. The test usually consists of five stages.

STAGE 1   Assessment of cash receipts
The consultant and family cash income will be assessed and quantified. This will typically consist of salary (net of income tax, national insurance and pension contributions), consultancy fees received in cash and other forms of payment, net of costs actually paid, and other income.

STAGE 2   Assessment of fixed identifiable cash payments
Typically, an individual's or a family's fixed cash payments will consist of monthly personal travel costs, mortgage, council tax, water rates, electricity and gas, household and contents insurance and telephone.

STAGE 3   Assessment of variable identifiable cash payments
Every consultant has a different variable lifestyle. The technique involves an assessment of annual expenditure on variable living costs, such as food and drink, clothing, consumables, motor vehicles, school fees and holidays. Frequently there is strong evidence available, as such expenses are paid by cheque or with credit cards.

STAGE 4   Assessment of variable unidentifiable cash payments
Many items of expenditure in an individual's or family's lifestyle are not specifically recorded. These include, for example, costs of entertaining, external eating and dining, gambling, church donations and family gifts. In the life-style test, estimates are made for all items.

STAGE 5   Assessment

This stage involves a rigorous comparison of the sources of cash income against identifiable items of cash expenditure. Where there is imbalance (i.e. recorded expenditure exceeding income or vice versa) to the trained inspector there may be undeclared income on which tax is due. The immediate presumption is that the consultant tax payer is guilty until proved innocent.

Penalties

The penalties on tax due on undeclared income, or overdeclared, non-allowable expenditure are now severe, even if innocent offences have been made. There are three types of penalty:

1. Interest. If additional tax is due following an enquiry, interest will be charged at commercial rates from the normal filing date of the tax return. These rates are varied from time to time.

2. Fixed penalties. A consultant tax payer may be subject to fixed penalty fines. These are currently £100 if a tax return is not filed by a due date; £200 if the return is not submitted within six months of the due date and, with the approval of the General or Special Commissioners, a fixed penalty of £60 per day on the day after a fixed penalty notice is served. There are special penalties of £50 plus £30 per day if documents are not supplied by a consultant for audit or discovery purposes. This can be increased to £150 per day, subject to General or Special Commissioner approval. Finally, the Revenue has powers to impose a penalty of up to £3000 in the event that a consultant has not retained his or her records in a proper fashion.

3. Variable penalties. Variable penalties of up to 100% tax payable can be imposed on a consultant if:

   – he or she has not received an appropriate tax return and, where there is tax payable, has not told the Revenue by 6 October following the financial year

   – the submission of the tax return is delayed by more than 12 months

– a tax return or accounts contain negligent or fraudulent errors or omissions. It should be noted that, in the Revenue's view even apparently innocent errors can be treated as 'fraudulent' and penalised accordingly.

Tax investigation insurance policies

Given the changes accompanying the introduction of the self assessment system, the stated Revenue objective of increasing investigating activity and the nature of many consultants' practices, risks of investigation are far higher than they were previously.

There are a number of insurance policies on the market that can offer a consultant some protection against the professional costs of investigation by the Revenue, the Contributions Agency and HM Customs and Excise. These can be effected individually through a reputable broker, or collectively. Costs of such policies are generally competitive and are recommended for the majority of consultants in practice.

As with all insurance policies, it is frequently the question of what is *not* covered by the policy that is relevant. For most tax investigations protection policies available to medical practitioners the following exclusions apply:

- cost of tax payable, including fines, penalties and interest

- any claim involving criminal proceedings instituted by the Revenue authorities

- costs arising from investigation of accounts and returns already submitted to the Revenue

- any matters existing at the date a policy is effective which a consultant ought *reasonably* to have known would give rise to a claim

- costs of any investigations that have arisen prior to the date of insurance

- any claim that involves use of published 'tax avoidance schemes'

- costs of dealing with the 'special officers' of the Inland Revenue. Such investigations are generally of a very serious nature and may involve suspected criminal activity

- any disputes or investigations where the chances of success are considered by the insurers to be very remote. In addition, most policies normally exclude the costs of making good any deficiencies to a consultant's books, records, accounts and returns and also costs of not complying with relevant legislation.

How to complain about the Revenue

While a considerable portion of this chapter has focused on the need for a consultant in practice to comply fully with the disciplines of the self assessment system, and the possible consequences if he or she does not do so, the Revenue is not omnipotent. There are an increasing number of areas of dispute between taxpayers and the Revenue as a result of mistakes and errors. Principal areas identified in the 1997 Official Adjudicators Report include cases where the tax inspector is confrontational and behaves in an unprofessional manner; where he or she is inconsistent in decision making; where there are delays in dealing with a tax payer's affairs; where poor tactics are employed in tax collection procedures; where the tax inspector does not clearly state the extent of his or her powers; where the tax inspector's own communication or record-keeping is poor, and where the tax inspector breaches confidentiality.

Specific recent examples of such behaviour in the medical sector have included:

- the problem of unnecessarily long investigations, which have carried considerable personal distress and worry to consultants and their families

- county court judgments for alleged unpaid tax incorrectly being assessed

- bankruptcy proceedings commencing for inaccurate or incomplete tax assessments, notwithstanding that information has been supplied to the Revenue

- poor advice from a Revenue Office, resulting in a consultant having a higher tax bill than appropriate

- discourtesy on the part of Revenue officials to a consultant, both personally or in correspondence.

If a consultant is dissatisfied with his or her treatment from the Revenue, the first step is to complain to the local manager or District Inspector either directly or through an agent. The Revenue has its own code of practice, 'Mistakes by the Inland Revenue', which allows it to make consolatory payments for worry and distress it may have caused in making serious errors.

The majority of complaints is settled in this way. If there is still no resolution, a consultant is entitled to file a complaint with the Official Adjudicators Office, located at 28 Haymarket, London SW1Y 4SP. This office is free, impartial and accessible, and has an increasing reputation for sorting out complaints satisfactorily.

8

Practice advisors

Successful businesses run as a team, with professional advisors very much part of the organisation. For most successful private practices the accountant, the solicitor and the financial advisor are part of that team. However, many consultants perform the roles of these professionals themselves in their businesses, with varying degrees of effectiveness. By doing so, they frequently make errors, miss opportunities and waste time that could be utilised to exploit their own particular skills and talents.

The accountant

The accountant is not infrequently perceived as someone who prepares accounts and tax returns at the end of the financial year and who plays a very limited role in the business. A good accountant, with honed financial and business management skills, can add a considerable element to a consultant's business. A poor accountant can do the opposite. Regrettably, the poor quality of much accounting work was commented on in the 1997 Adjudicator's Report. References were made to examples of poor work and communication by some accountants, a lack of technical knowledge in dealing with their clients' affairs, a confrontational attitude by the accountant towards the Revenue, charging excessive fees in dealing particularly with tax matters and plain wrong-doing by the accountant in collaboration with, or independent of the client.

Sadly, the choice of accountant by many medical clients is made on the basis of cost alone, rather than on the basis of the incremental benefit that the advisor can bring to the consultant business over his or her costs. Good accountants are in demand and their costs reflect their skills and value. While professional bodies and advertising material can assist in the choice of any accountant, for most medical practitioners, word of mouth or reputation should be the two key factors influencing initial choices. Frequently, an individual accountant may be an appropriate first choice for an individual consultant. While many large accounting firms have exceptional skills, their costs and overhead structure are such that a small consultant's business can probably only be serviced at a very junior level.

Consultants do have the ability to manage their financial advice costs, though many commit business errors, which ensure that their accountancy fees are perhaps higher than they could be. Common errors are listed below.

ERROR 1 Have no book-keeping system
Despite the current tax system with its emphasis on records, a minority of consultants operates extremely poor record systems. Lack of invoices, payment records, banking and reconciliation systems offer an accountant the chance to charge fees merely to sort things out. Internal procedures and book-keeping systems adequately operated can reduce the expensive nature of reconstruction fees.

ERROR 2 Fall out with your bank manager
Those consultants regularly in trouble with their bankers risk facing potentially larger accounting fees. Bank managers can, and do, demand up-to-date accountants' reports, projections and interim accounts. Such 'emergency' type work carries a premium. Those consultants who ensure that their bank manager is well informed (Chapter 6) can avoid such fees.

ERROR 3 Choose a non-specialist accountant
Accountancy is still a profession where generalism prevails. In

medicine, specialism is now commonplace. While most accountants have to know the basic taxation and accounting rules there are special industry knowledge requirements. General accountants without such knowledge are often on a learning curve when they are dealing with specialist private practice problems. Inevitably the costs of learning are not infrequently passed on to the client.

ERROR 4   Choose a non-qualified accountant
The accountancy profession in the UK still operates under six separate 'chartered' bodies. In addition, there are a number of other reputable accountancy support and book-keeping professional bodies. There is no overriding professional body such as the BMA that can coordinate the interests and services of qualified accountants. Consequently the market contains a large number of unqualified individuals who are able to practice as 'accountants'. The quality of service provided by such individuals varies from excellent to dreadful. Some unqualified accountants practice without any indemnity insurance or professional control. They are therefore able to offer a relatively cheap service. Experience in all walks of life shows that people receive what they pay for. Unqualified cheap service is often a panacea for future problems.

ERROR 5   Don't ask the cost of accountancy services
Accountants are in business to sell their time. The more time that is sold, the higher their incomes. However, accountants do operate in a competitive market and will accept readily requests for quotes for work from medical clients. Frequently accountants' costs are reduced where a medical client opts to place his business on a 'job quote' rather than on 'a time cost' basis.

ERROR 6   'Leave everything to the accountant'
Some medical consultants leave everything to their accountant, presenting him or her at the end of a financial year with a box full of disorganised files and papers. Sorting files and papers is expensive. Detective work costs a client money, which is legitimately charged by the accountant if the client has no immediate and ready explanation.

ERROR 7   Be reluctant to consider change

Some years ago, medical businesses often regarded their professional advisors as partners for life. Technical progress, changes in the way the profession operates and a more competitive market are all factors in encouraging a more fluid approach to a relationship. Frequently a medical client moving to a new accountant can negotiate a reduction in accountancy fees. Some accountants do offer 'introductory' fee packages. However, it is important to remember that a good, stable relationship, where the accountant knows the medical client's business well and can advise accordingly is often preferable to a climate of constant revolution and change, where advice may be given with less understanding of the history.

ERROR 8   Be reluctant to complain

Accountants are human and do make mistakes, despite the fact that most attempt to provide a professional service to their client. In most cases mistakes will be corrected and the client fees reduced accordingly. In other instances, the accountant may not be aware of an error or problem. A complaint by a consultant is frequently appropriate. A professional accountant will be anxious to ensure that any loss to their client is minimised and will take steps to ensure that matters are solved equitably. Those clients who fester their complaints and concerns are doing themselves, their business and their relationship with their accountant no good whatsoever.

ERROR 9   Do everything yourself

As indicated above, some medical consultants do everything themselves to save fees and expense. Mistakes are not uncommon: medical income may be undeclared; more frequently, consultants do not claim for all expenses or allowances to which they are reasonably entitled. As indicated in Chapter 7, the cost of making mistakes in accounts and tax returns can now be extremely high. To rely on untrained accountancy skills may, in the long term, be expensive.

ERROR 10   Ignore computerisation

The question of information systems was considered in Chapter 4. Appropriate computerisation is an important factor in operating an efficient private practice. Good accountants can assist their clients in this respect. Computerised records, well prepared, provide appreciably better base information with which to prepare accounts than the traditional box. As a result, costs will reduce. Those consultants in private practice who remain devoted to historical book-keeping systems and who ignore computerisation will face a spiral of rising accountancy costs.

It is important to recognise that cost pressures are affecting all industries and professions. Private medical practitioners have been comparatively late in recognising that they are able to influence costs of their accountancy services and at the same time to enjoy an increased standard of service. Those who do recognise this and find the right accountant for them, will find that they are better able to offload the financial pressures, problems and statutory requirements on to someone who is technically and professionally able – at a competitive price.

The solicitor

In the private medical practice, a solicitor can have two major roles. First, the lawyer can offer a protective service to ensure that all matters in the practice are appropriately dealt with. Second, he or she can offer a mediation, conciliation or, if appropriate, a litigation service.

Much of what has been said about the choice of an accountant for the practice is appropriate to the solicitor. Word of mouth, reputation and, for many in private practice, members of small quality firms with some industry knowledge are pre-requisite.

The legal audit

Ignoring professional negligence claims, private medical practice businesses frequently face a common range of legal problems:

- debt collection problems
- employment disputes with staff

- contractual disputes

- Inland Revenue investigations

- breaches of the Health and Safety Act

- breaches of restrictive covenants

- for those trading as a limited liability company, breaches of the various Companies Acts.

Legal costs can often become high as a result of litigation where there is defective, inadequate or non-existent legal documentation.

A primary function of a proactive legal advisor to the private medical practice is to ensure that all documentation is in order, appropriately updated, and that the business complies with all the various statutes pertaining to it. This can be achieved through the so-called legal audit process, where all documentation is reviewed and, if appropriate, updated. For large practices, an annual review is often cost-effective. For smaller businesses, this review can be biennial or triannual. A checklist of the types of matter typically covered in such an audit is given in Appendix B. While it is not comprehensive, it illustrates the large number of legal matters that even the smallest private medical practice has to consider. As with accounting records, regular review and maintenance of this documentation can reduce potential problems at a later stage.

Litigation

One of the major unexpected costs facing a consultant in private practice is the cost of litigation. There is an inextricable trend towards more litigation in the medical sector. People suggest that the UK is already experiencing the unseemly American spectacle of lawyers chasing ambulances and searching hospital wards and patient waiting rooms for business. There are examples of solicitors setting up local offices at NHS hospitals. The proposed phasing out of legal aid and the introduction of 'no win – no fee' cases is opening up new areas of business for litigation lawyers.

As the first and obvious line of defence, all in private practice need to ensure that their compulsory professional indemnity and negligence insurance is adequate and appropriate for the nature of their business. Insurance rates from leading insurers such as the Medical Defence Union depend, for example, on the nature of the medical business insured and the volume of fees generated. Compulsory insurance cover should be reviewed at least annually (particularly for the growing practice) and expert advice should be taken if in doubt. There is still a minority of consultants in practice who do not have full cover. They are taking a large and unnecessary risk.

Where insurers are involved in any legal action, they will generally handle the conduct of matters. In dealing with litigation lawyers (whether insured or not), a number of simple steps needs to be taken by consultants to minimise their costs. Those unfortunate enough to have become involved in litigation of any kind, including divorce, will know that legal fees can become a never-ending continuum. The basic steps in managing litigation fees are to:

- agree with the lawyer the precise objective of the litigation

- agree with the lawyer a brief and plan of action

- agree with the lawyer a timetable

- agree with the lawyer a cost budget. Ask to be informed if, at any time, costs exceed the budget

- agree, in advance, the basis of charging and what is to be charged for

- agree if there is any 'no win – no fee' element

- monitor at all times the progress of litigation on both an achievement and a cost basis

- make *prompt* comments and/or criticism if there are variations of any kind to the initial agreed course of action

- ask for a detailed breakdown of invoices when raised. Failure to query bills early may result in problems at a later stage

- agree in advance a plan of action if there is unhappiness or discontent with the lawyer's actions. Consultants sometimes do, primarily through inertia, remain with an inactive or ineffective lawyer. A lack of confidence can be expensive.

Finally, it should be noted that the legal professional is still steeped in a tradition of billing against a code of conduct not widely disseminated. The rules controlling lawyers' bills are made by lawyers. Managing legal costs in the same way that consultants manage other costs in their businesses and private lives can save money and ensure that they receive value for money. Litigation of any kind is expensive, and without tight management those consultants unfortunate enough to be involved stand the risk of significant financial loss or, in the ultimate, ruin.

The independent financial advisor

As a result of their high earnings relative to the rest of the community, consultants in private practice are a prime target for salesmen of financial products, including life assurance, disability insurance, term insurance, pensions and the range of financial instruments available in the market. These salesmen originate from the banks, possibly their accountants and their solicitors, their professional organisations, financial services groups and from many other private sources.

There are a large number of consultants who have been tempted by a range of different financial products purchased at different times. Many have an uncoordinated 'mish-mash' of products. Central to the financial products salesmen's interest in medical consultants is the high potential commission earnings available.

It is, of course, incumbent on the prudent individual in private medical practice to plan his or her financial affairs and to purchase an appropriate range of financial products to protect him or herself and family against death or serious illness. A good independent financial advisor can assist greatly in this process. While the choice of advisor is very much one of individual consultant's preference the more professional financial advisors will:

- not be 'tied' to any particular insurance or other company and will therefore be able to advise generally on a range of products

- be prepared to undertake a full appraisal of the consultant's financial position and objectives. While such 'fact finds' are now obligatory under the Financial Services legislation, the quality of research varies considerably

- be prepared to discuss alternative strategies with the consultant's other advisors, notably his accountant and solicitor

- readily disclose commission terms relating to any products. Again, this should be obligatory under current legislation, but some financial advisors are less forthcoming than others

- be prepared to work for a fixed fee, with all commission, both immediate and future, being added back to the financial product to the benefit of the consultants

- have had a fairly stable career and will have not worked for a wide range of different firms and organisations.

Other professionals will of course be part of a consultant's line of advisors at varying stages of their business career. However, strong, competent and trustworthy accountants, solicitors and financial advisors are critical to long-term business success.

9

Relationships with the NHS

It is not the purpose of this book to discuss the operations and management of the NHS other than in so far as it affects a consultant in the development of his or her private practice.

The climate of ongoing change and rationing

At the time of writing, the service is still considering the implications of the 1997 White Paper, 'The New NHS: Modern Dependable'. This represents the new Labour Governments' policy for the future of the NHS. Ideas and concepts have been borrowed from the previous Government's White Paper, 'Working for Change'. A good analysis of the implications of the 1997 White Paper is given in Mark Baker's book, *Making Sense of the New NHS White Paper*.[1]

Many consultants are cynical of the ongoing changes made to the operations, management and philosophy of their primary employer. They have become disillusioned as to the value of paperwork and their changing role from being the director to the plumber or artisan. This ongoing disillusionment may be a fundamental reason why so many seek the apparently calmer

[1] Baker M (1998) *Making Sense of the New NHS White Paper*. Radcliffe Medical Press, Oxford.

waters, with less political interference, of private practice. The latest White Paper perhaps gives no solace to those with this view. Neither does it give comfort to those who believe that the NHS is under a process, in business terms, of secular long-term decline. While the 1997 White Paper and 1998 Department of Health announcements promise further cash to the service, consultants in the front line are still seeing the problems of rationing, inequality and the holding down of the pay of professional staff.

Despite the politicians' fine words, this present situation is likely to continue. In 1998, for example, the Institute of Fiscal Studies has concluded that the future growth in the demand for public health services will be greater than that of its ability to supply. As a result, ongoing and increased rationing of services is likely to continue. There appears to be no realistic option other than a continuation of the status quo. Ongoing frustration for many consultants will not be removed by the Government's latest initiatives.

From a business point of view to the individual consultant, the 1997 White Paper perhaps introduces two further opportunities for professional recognition and furtherance. This is through the proposed establishment of the National Institute for Clinical Excellence (the so-called NICE) and the Commission for Health Improvements (the so-called CHIMP). The principal stated objectives of NICE, which is intended to operate under the auspices of the professional Royal Colleges, are to:

- provide a forum to give new coherence and prominence to information about clinical- and cost-effectiveness

- produce and disseminate clinical guidelines based on relevant evidence of clinical- and cost-effectiveness

- produce and disseminate clinical audit methodologies and information on good practice in clinical audit.

The stated objectives of CHIMP are to support and oversee the quality of clinical governance and of clinical services.

The benefit to the individual consultant if these two proposed bodies become effectively operational, is that there will be some independent audit and a comparative database against which his or her own performance can be monitored. This could provide, if relevant, for major marketing opportunities in the private practice of 'product performance'. At present, however, this option is still probably some years ahead.

Employment contracts with the NHS

The vast majority of consultants in the UK relies on the NHS as its primary source of income. Perhaps fewer than 500 work entirely in the private sector. Their contract with the NHS, and its precise wording, can help or hinder their ability to establish and develop a private practice.

There are, in essence, three types of contract which a consultant can typically enter into with the NHS.

1. A whole- or full-time contract. Under such a contract, a consultant contracts with the NHS for 'substantially the whole of their professional time'. In conventional terms, however, this is not necessarily akin to full-time employment. This is because consultant days in the NHS are divided into so-called notional half days (NHDs) of $3\frac{1}{2}$ hours each, to be worked flexibly. The theory is that 10 NHDs equate to a week's work. A consultant with a whole-time contract is allowed to work in private practice, subject to a restriction that gross income from this source does not exceed 10% of his or her salary, including merit award. Most NHS trusts have procedures whereby whole-time consultants have to certify, on an annual basis, that their income from private practice does not exceed 10% of their NHS income. Many trusts have powers to call for accounts and records to support the claim, but surprisingly, few appear to do so. They also have powers to convert a consultant's contract from a whole-time to a maximum part-time basis, if circumstances show this to be appropriate.

2. A maximum part-time contract. This contract basis seems to be the most popular for many consultants who have a desire to develop seriously their private practice. Under the terms of such a contract there are no restrictions on the amount of income from private practice that can be earned. However, under such a contract, a consultant still has to devote 'substantially the whole

of his professional time to the NHS'. This involves working a minimum of 10 NHDs. However, in view of the lack of restrictions on private income earning ability, a consultant under this contract type receives only 10/11 of the equivalent whole-time salary and award package.

3. A part-time contract. Under such a contract a consultant does not have to offer a 'substantial' proportion of his or her time to the NHS. He or she can work between one and nine NHDs per week, each NHD generating 1/11 of the whole-time consultant's salary. Under such a contract, there are no restrictions on private practice.

The policing of the three alternative types of contract still appears to be surprisingly lax. The BMA does require its members to 'observe the spirit of the rules'. However, in practice there is little effective formal monitoring and the system is open to exploitation. For example:

- whole-time contract holders can exceed their 10% earnings rule

- consultants on maximum part-time contracts can easily breach their commitment and devote more time to private practice

- consultants on part-time contracts can easily abuse their contractual commitment to the NHS.

It is, regrettably, generally up to the individual consultant to determine whether he or she does or does not neglect NHS duties.

Category One and Category Two work

Many new consultants are surprisingly ignorant as to what exactly is defined as 'private practice' work. The formal definition, contained in the general 'Terms and Conditions of Service of Hospital, Medical and Dental Staff' is not helpful. This document defines 'private practice' as 'the diagnosis and treatment of patients by private arrangement'. A 'private patient' is defined as 'one who has given an undertaking to pay for both accommodation and medical services'.

Under most NHS consultant contracts, there are, in fact, three types of work.

Category One work

Such work is defined as the 'diagnosis and treatment of NHS patients'. This definition is reasonably straightforward.

Category Two work

This is fee-paid work that consultants are permitted to undertake in conjunction with NHS work without restriction, notwithstanding their contract type. In general terms, Category Two work does *not* include direct treatment of patients. It can include, for example, examinations and reports prepared for various non-NHS purposes, such as for courts, the police, and for social security and insurance benefits. Illustrative lists of Category Two work are included in the 'Terms and Conditions of Service of Hospital, Medical and Dental Staff'.

There are, of course, opportunities for consultants to undertake Category Two work that will not bring them into conflict with their employment contract. The availability of Category Two work can often allow a young consultant to establish his or her private practice at an early stage, without any of the inherent risks or potential loss of incomes resulting from a change of contract type. However, evidence suggests that long-term income opportunities for Category Two work are not generally substantial. They can be time-consuming and can detract from seeking more profitable private work. Where a consultant does, however, use NHS facilities to enable him or her to undertake such work, the normal arrangement is for one third of fees received to be remitted to the provider of facilities. Generally, the consultant will have to pay directly, in addition, for secretarial and administrative support services. It should be noted that some NHS trusts, however, do seek to ensure that all income from Category Two work is reimbursed fully.

Private practice work

This work is as defined above. Conduct of such work is subject to the contractual constraints imposed by the elected employment contract.

Negotiation of NHS contracts

The health service reforms introduced by the last Conservative Government in conjunction with local shortages of specialist skills have opened up opportunities for the consultant as businessman. This is through the precise negotiation of his contractual basis of employment with the NHS. Sadly, many consultants merely accept what is on offer once they are offered the chance of a consultancy. However, evidence shows that many NHS trusts are prepared to show flexibility in attracting and retaining key staff. Professional attention to negotiation of an NHS contract can enhance income earning potential from employment and allow opportunity for development of a private practice. The inherent restrictions of many NHS consultants' contracts have, in turn, led to the establishment of feeble private practice businesses.

Consultants negotiating contracts with their NHS employers are in the same position as people seeking employment in any sector. Four basic steps can maximise success from an employment negotiation.

1. Identification, in advance of the precise business goals of the consultant. What, for example, does he or she hope to achieve from NHS employment? What is his or her attitude towards private practice?

2. The undertaking of detailed market research. Those consultants who have researched the national and local market for their specialties and their costs and in particular have researched any potential local shortages are frequently better able to negotiate an improved package for themselves.

3. Preparation of an employment 'wish list' in advance. It is a fairly obvious statement, but a clear view of employment requirements can often reap benefits.

4. Identification of an employment/private practice action plan in advance of interview. Consultants who intend to develop a private practice do need to consider, in some detail, exactly how NHS employment can assist them in development of their future practice. For example, advantages of employment with a particu-

lar trust can include the contact base, the potential research facilities and the availability of a local market. It should be noted that there are professional employment consultants who can assist a consultant in preparation for interview and a negotiating package. An investment in this area can often reap rewards.

Content of employment contract

Given the increased flexibility resulting from the establishment of trusts, it is possible to negotiate more flexible contracts than was the case perhaps ten years ago. Typical features that need to be covered are:

- job title
- job description
- dates of commencement and assessment of 'continuing employment' provisions
- normal place of work. It is increasingly important that this is defined properly for tax reasons
- basis of pay and remuneration
- period of payment
- normal hours and arrangements, if any, for overtime and anti-social hours
- holiday entitlement provisions
- procedures in the event of absence for sickness and/or other reasons
- pension entitlement. NHS pension arrangements are now very complex, and professional advice from an independent financial advisor or accountant (see Chapter 8) should normally be sought before agreeing to any pension arrangements
- provisions as to notice. In particular, it is important to understand the provisions in respect of termination of employment by both the employer and the employee

- provisions as to normal retirement

- provisions as to reimbursement of travel and other expenses

- provisions for training and ongoing professional education

- for consultants starting in a new position, provision and policy in relation to relocation expenses. Experience has shown that consultants' relocation expenses can be treated either in a tax efficient or a tax inefficient manner unless properly negotiated

- disciplinary rules and suspension procedures

- grievance procedures.

While the employment negotiations procedure is typically considered only when a consultant is changing positions, it should be noted that contracts of employment can be amended at any time. A healthy ongoing review process of employment contracts can ensure that a consultant's personal objectives vis-à-vis employment and private practice can be fully maintained and reconciled.

The 'whistle blowing' phenomenon

It has been indicated above that, in practice, control and audit of a consultant's behaviour in relation to performance of his or her contract is at best random. While the majority of consultants do follow their professional bodies' advice and 'stick to the spirit' of contracted arrangements there are notable exceptions and examples of abuse.

In recent months, there has been both directly and anonymously an increasing political climate and encouragement of 'whistle blowing'. By this is meant a reporting to the authorities of consultants who appear to be operating outside the terms of their contracts. The theory is laudable, but in practice, official encouragement of 'whistle blowing' will encourage a number of potentially sinister developments. For example:

- the reporting of consultants to management by staff who, for whatever reason, hold some kind of grudge against them

- the reporting of consultants to other bodies, either directly or more frequently anonymously. Most notably reports are sometimes made to the Inland Revenue or to medical insurance companies. These bodies do investigate reports, whether made maliciously or otherwise

- the circulation of anonymous material, perhaps with some element of truth, which can damage a consultant's reputation or business.

It is likely that 'whistle blowing' as a phenomenon will increase and will affect perfectly innocent consultants. It should be noted that under the terms of the Public Interest Disclosure Act, which came into force in December 1998, an employee who legitimately 'whistle blows' will be protected from retaliatory action by an employer. This Act will probably have the effect of increasing the extent of malicious 'whistle blowing'. It can cause disruption, stress and generally a not insignificant cost to rectify matters. The common sense advice is for all consultants to recognise this phenomenon and to conduct their affairs appropriately. Adequate documentation is the most common defence to claims, both spurious or otherwise. Those few who do abuse the rules flagrantly will, in time, be penalised.

Use of NHS facilities by consultants for their private practice

For consultants starting work in private practice, NHS facilities are an obvious first choice. This is particularly the case if they have not established a sufficiently strong contact network to enable them to establish themselves in private hospitals. Other consultants with mature businesses use 'pay beds' in NHS hospitals as a first priority.

The attitude towards 'pay beds' by various hospitals still varies. However, the majority of hospitals recognise the propensity for additional income resulting from private use of beds by patients and seek, implicitly or explicitly, to encourage this activity.

For those consultants who consider the option of admitting patients to NHS beds (and the majority should), it is important to be aware of a number of factors.

- Under the 1998 Health and Medicines Act, local hospitals are empowered to establish their own charges to accommo- dation, theatre time, staff costs, etc. A consultant in private practice should be fully conversant with local NHS hospital charges.

- Consultants using NHS pay beds should be aware of the so- called 'Green Book' published in 1986 and revised in 1993 (officially known as 'The guide to the management of private practice in health service hospitals in England and Wales'). This book covers the procedures for handling private patients in NHS hospitals. It also describes, in some detail, the NHS philosophy that private patients should not have an unfair advantage over non-paying ones. The 'Green Book' acts as a good guide to the management of private patients in the NHS and should be in every consultant's library. There seems little point, therefore, in repeating the guidelines of the book in this forum.

However, one matter does deserve comment. This is the situation where a patient, following consultation, decides to change status from NHS to private. Where a patient elects to seek treatment in an independent hospital from where a consultant conducts private practice there is often little difficulty. Individual consultants can experience problems, however, where an NHS patient elects to become a private patient with treatment from an NHS hospital. There is often the suggestion that consultants are able to manipulate a patient's view, or permit him or her to act under duress. Such a move, if frequent, opens up scope for 'whistle blowing' and charges of professional misconduct. In this situation the consultant should take heed, particularly, of Clauses 22 through 27 of the original 1986 Green Book, which covers ethical and procedural implications of such a situation. Strict adherence to the advice in the Green Book can avoid the potential for problems.

The key decisions – when to opt out?

One of the most common questions asked by consultants of their accountants or business advisors, is when to 'opt out' of the NHS to concentrate on private practice. For many, this is merely a pipe dream, for the market evidence is that few actually take this step. Nonetheless, the apparent frustration of continuing employment in the late 1990s NHS causes many to consider this option.

Those consultants who have taken this step (as indicated above, probably fewer than 500 in the UK) have generally succeeded commercially. This is because their business talents, combined with their professional skills, have enabled them to develop their markets and to survive.

In practice, a large number of consultants should not even consider leaving the security of their NHS contract for the inherent insecurity of the marketplace. This is because of their own personal goal structure; lack of business experience and determination; feelings of instinctive insecurity, and concern at loss of a contract base and network structure. However, there is a not insignificant number of consultants who would benefit financially from working entirely in the private sector. For them the 'opt out' question is a reality.

A potential decision by a consultant to 'opt out' completely should only be made after the most vigorous and self-critical analysis covering:

- analysis of personal and family goals

- analysis of the existing NHS employment package and in particular accrued pension rights

- analysis of the growth and performance of their existing private practice

- analysis of how their private practice is currently generated

- analysis of the importance of the current NHS contact structure

- preparation of a business plan for a potential full-time private practice. This topic is considered more fully in Chapter 11

- analysis of taxation implications of any changes

- a full understanding of the potential loss to the business of NHS resources, both directly and indirectly.

Opting out is a brave decision. Market evidence does support the saying that 'who dares, wins', but pre-planning and careful analysis are essential.

10

The medical insurance companies

One of the most important practical business relationships for a consultant in private practice is with the medical insurance companies. Effectively they, rather than the patient, are the paymasters. The relationship can have significant implications for the commercial success or otherwise of a consultant in practice. An understanding of the history is important to the formulation by a consultant of his or her approach to the insurance companies.

The historical development of practice private medical insurance

To understand the market for private medical insurance (PMI) today it is helpful to know how it has developed since the Second World War.

Before the introduction of the NHS in 1948, the middle classes thought it prudent to save, through provident associations, a regular amount to defray the costs of private hospital treatment should this become necessary. GPs were paid a cash fee for services unless an individual was earning below a certain income level. In such cases it was possible to apply for assistance, with the result that GPs' costs were met by the local authority.

The provident system was based locally, and at the time of the inception of the NHS in 1948, it was thought that there would be no further need for such an arrangement. The provident associations came under the shelter of British United Provident Association (BUPA) in 1947, ostensibly to wind them up as the perceived need for them became less.

For about three years after the establishment of the NHS there was a decline in the number of private subscribers. However, as people realised that the NHS left a lot to be desired in terms of privacy, choice of consultant specialist and speed of delivery, particularly for non-urgent matters, the number of subscribers started to rise again. The NHS, at its formation, inherited a long waiting list.

There was steady growth in the number of private medical insurance subscribers throughout the 1950s and 60s and by the mid-1970s about five million people were covered by the provident associations. There was negligible interest from commercial insurers in this market. The two major providents, BUPA and PPP, covered most people, with many having their subscriptions paid for as a company 'perk'.

During the period, subscription income invariably exceeded claims, the difference being reinvested on behalf of the subscribers. As the number of subscribers continued to increase the insurers became worried about the availability of suitable nursing homes for private patients seeking elective surgery. As a result, BUPA was instrumental as early as the 1950s in setting up the Nuffield Nursing Home Trust (now Nuffield Hospitals) to cater for the increasing demand.

In the 1970s, elective surgery was still relatively simple. But the concept of 'replacement' was gathering momentum and coronary artery surgery was beginning to become recognised. Hysterectomy and prostate operations, however, were still usually carried out through abdominal incisions and required a 10-day postoperative stay in hospital. Subscribers to provident association policies usually tried the NHS first for these services as the independent hospitals did not provide facilities for highly complex surgery. As late as 1980, more than 80% of private hospitals work, was in the minor or intermediate category of surgery.

The Labour Government policies of the late 1970s

The first major change to this cosy situation of minor surgery in independent hospitals and innovative treatment in the NHS occurred when the Labour Government of the late 1970s attempted to eliminate private practice completely. History shows that the private sector fought back and survived. The outcome was, perhaps, not as politically envisaged and there were two major effects on the PMI market. First, there was rapid growth in the number of new subscribers, and second, these new subscribers began to use private facilities more. The incidence of insurance claims also started to rise.

Largely as a result of political pressures in the late 1970s, the private sector decided to reduce its dependence on the NHS and to build more sophisticated hospitals. These were specifically designed for safe, elective surgery of any complexity. This was an expensive task, partly because the private demand for medical services in a local area usually required hospitals with less than 100 beds, across which the capital costs had to be spread. This was reflected in the relatively high price of a day's hospital stay.

The 1980s experience

Following the changes above, commercial medical operators entered the medical market for the first time. American money was used in the 1980s to finance one of the largest chains of independent hospitals. BUPA also decided to invest a high proportion of its reserves in healthcare facilities. As a result of these decisions, BUPA hospitals are one of the largest providers of private hospital care today.

Commercial insurers, seeing what appeared to be a growth market for medical insurance in the 1980s, also arrived. These often had the backing of large insurance companies with high reserves and they started to erode the traditional market of the provident. New commercial insurers introduced concepts from other areas of the insurance industry, such as 'no claims bonuses' and 'excess' payments into private medical health insurance. They sold their policies through established chains of brokers paying commissions. Up to that time, such a move would have been thought unthinkable.

Contemporaneously in the 1980s, surgical techniques – to deal with coronary artery disease, joint and lens replacement – and through the endoscope, had progressed rapidly. The proportion of people living until an age when these surgical procedures really did improve their quality of life was increasing dramatically. As a result of these socioeconomic factors the incidence of claims also continued to rise until late into the decade.

Insurance companies in the 1990s

As a result of these changes, the medical insurance business arrived at the recession of the 1990s in a very volatile state. A number of factors was significant.

- First, premiums had been rising rapidly in the 1980s to counteract the increase in claims and the cost of a more independent private sector. The newly arrived commercial insurers often underwrote business at a loss to tempt subscribers away from the traditional provident associations. Commercial business organisations, which were responsible for paying around 60% of subscribed premiums at the beginning of the 1990s, were insisting on keeping overall costs down. Commercial business was also increasingly questioning insurers about the extent of quality assessment they were making on their providers of services.

- Second, the building of independent hospitals continued, often concentrating on providing beds when, in fact, average length of stay was falling and day surgery was rising in popularity.

- Third, changes in the NHS in the early 1990s did give an incentive to trust managers to improve their own provision of private beds. By the mid-1990s there was therefore a surplus of beds in the independent sector. A free market economist might have expected the price of a night in hospital to have fallen, but the medical market did not respond in this way.

The effect of the Monopolies and Mergers Commission report

The market pressures to reduce consultants' costs was, perhaps, one fundamental reason for the investigation into private fees by the Monopolies and Mergers Commission (MMC). In 1992, the MMC declared that the BMA schedule of fees for private procedures was anticompetitive. The BMA subsequently withdrew its list. However, the MMC ruled that schedules drawn up by insurance companies relating to a particular insurance plan were not anticompetitive. The oldest of these – the BUPA scheme – has, surprisingly, not been significantly updated since that time.

The 1992 report has had a significant impact on consultants' pricing. Some consultants have even kept their prices for procedures at their 1992 level. They, however, charged significantly more for consultations and the practice of 'unbundling' has started to increase. This is discussed later in the chapter.

The current situation

Today, the market for health insurance has declined slightly from its peak in the late 1980s. However, more people are paying for private medicine out of their own pockets and, as a result, activity in the private sector is still buoyant. However, no medical insurance company of any size is believed to be making a profit on its premium income.

The insurance companies remain solvent from their investment income, support from their owners and, in BUPA's case, from the profits of their hospital and overseas activities. As a result, there is continuing pressure by insurance companies to control or manage consultancy fees charged through such means, for example, as 'managed care'.

Current medical insurance policies

In the current market, both patients and consultants in private practice are faced with a bewildering array of medical insurance policies. Since the arrival in the market of the commercial operators in the late 1980s, and the demands made by client companies for tailored products, the types of policy available are legion.

The majority of medical insurance policies is designed to cover 'acute medical conditions' only. That statement, in itself, is ambiguous, as the definitions of 'acute', 'medical' and 'condition' can all be reasonably questioned. Essentially, the overall definition means medical or surgical conditions for which there is a reasonably quick solution.

It is important that consultants recognise, at all times, what exactly is covered by their patients' policies. There are often anomalies. PMI policies will, for example, cover the diagnosis and investigation of diabetes, but will not cover long-term regular attendance at a diabetic clinic. They will often cover hip replacement surgery for osteoarthritis, but will not cover regular attendance at a rheumatology clinic for someone with chronic rheumatoid arthritis. Paradoxically, many policies cover interventional procedures for acute exacerbations of rheumatoid arthritis.

The importance of understanding excluded conditions before treatment

There has to be some starting point for any PMI policy before which existing disease is not covered, otherwise sick people would take out insurance and quickly bankrupt the system. This would be like taking out house insurance after the fire had started. The existence of disease is often extracted from a form completed by applicants, in which they state their medical history. This form is scrutinised by the insurer, who then excludes certain conditions from the policy. Consultants need to understand the nature of exclusion before commencing private treatment. Some insurers do not require subscribers to supply a medical history, but in the event of a claim they retrospectively examine GPs' records for evidence that the condition was pre-existing. In such policies there may be a moratorium condition which excludes treatment of pre-existing conditions for the first two years of the policy.

It is important for consultants in practice to note that most PMI policies do not cover cosmetic surgery, normal pregnancy, most dental procedures, palliative and terminal care. Many policies also exclude diseases related to alcoholism, drug abuse and AIDS. Regrettably, conditions attached to policies change frequently, and consultants who are not aware of the extent of their patients' true cover can suffer.

There will occasionally be controversy over exclusions, particularly in determining the distinction between 'acute' and 'chronic' disease. For example, where removal of normal breast tissue cures backache, rather than being a purely cosmetic procedure; where a pregnancy is 'normal'; or whether treatment of leukaemia with chemotherapy is palliative or curative. Such controversies are adjudicated first by senior non-medical people in the claims department of an insurance company, and second, by a medical adviser employed by the company. If controversy remains, then in most cases application can be made to the Insurance Ombudsman. Ultimately, the courts may decide, but this is a very rare event. The medical insurance industry deals with something like 12 000 claims per working day and there are only a handful of court cases pending.

Where there is controversy a consultant has, to all intents and purposes, to fight his patient's corner. Good documentation, sound analysis and an understanding of the precise wording of the insurance policy is essential.

In addition to medical exclusions, there are a number of different insurance policies on the market for different eventualities. A consultant in practice needs to be aware of the limitation of cover of those policies. For example, a cheaper policy than the normal comprehensive one covers a subscriber where the NHS waiting list for a particular condition is greater than a given number of weeks. This is commonly referred to as a 'six-week policy'. As it is unusual for any patient with suspected cancer to have to wait six weeks even for an NHS appointment, these policies can generally be considered to exclude treatment for cancer.

Other policies will only cover outpatient treatment. Some policies provide for referral to an alternative practitioner, but in such cases the subscriber must usually be referred by a GP. Most policies do not, however, cover outpatient medication or appliances.

Published price schedules

Most insurers publish a schedule of what they would expect to pay for a given procedure. The common classification of procedures is based loosely on the Office of Populations Census and Statistics coding system. This system was designed to measure hospital activity and for this purpose clinicians were often encouraged to list all the items that contributed to a procedure. When modified for billing purposes, the schedule price takes account of the fact that a procedure may consist of a number of minor procedures. The insurance company standard rules are that these should not be coded. For example, the quoted fee code for transurethral resection of the prostate (TURP) includes an element of cystoscopy, which is invariably part of the procedure. The fee for abdominal hysterectomy includes oophrectomy. Both cystoscopy and oophrectomy have codes in their own right and are sometimes listed with the major procedure on specialist bills, thereby inflating the fee.

This practice is called 'unbundling' in the USA, where it is fraudulent. In Britain, it is becoming increasingly common, presumably in response to the fact that there has been no major review of specialist fees for the last five years. It is, however, still not widespread. The knock-on effect of unbundling is that creative hospital accountants, in addition to consultants, attempt to increase the hospital bill by adding supplementary procedures. They are often able to justify their actions by the fact that the consultant has put it on his or her bill. Through this process it is possible to inflate the theatre, drugs and dressings charges, even though no extra equipment has been used.

Insurance company claims examiners are trained in the art of spotting unbundling and now seem to 'unbundle' claims. They are aware of consultants who follow such procedures and, in the extreme, can seek to take punitive action.

Preferred providers

Most insurance policies define a 'specialist' as a registered medical practitioner who holds, or has held, a consultant appointment within the NHS. There is little further check. Over the years, however, there has been considerable publicity about operations and procedures which have gone wrong. This has led to the business sector asking health insurers what quality assurance schemes they have in place to protect their own subscribers from negligent practices. This demand has led to some insurers applying their own criteria to clinical matters. In this way they are attempting to control the medical or surgical process, ostensibly to assure quality, but with a hope that costs will also be contained.

The medical profession has been very slow to react to these initiatives by the insurance industry. Only recently have the Royal Colleges started to make public their thoughts and activities on the concept of medical audit. It is, of course, very difficult to guarantee quality in statistical terms in the independent medical sector. Postoperative mortality is very rare, mostly because the patients are carefully selected and are undergoing low-risk, elective surgery. Very little follow-up and postoperative assessment is carried out in the private sector and, because the proportion of work is small, compared to most specialists' NHS practices, the figures are statistically insignificant. However, there is no doubt that individual insurance companies would like to contract with a much smaller proportion of the medical profession than they do at present. There is a strong possibility that over the next 10 years the concept of 'preferred providers' will develop. 'Preferred providers' are those specialists who are prepared to submit their practice to scrutiny and act within recognised guidelines. For such control, they may receive slightly enhanced fees. The first attempts of insurance companies in the mid-1990s to introduce the concept of 'preferred providers' have not been a success. At the time of writing, relationships between consultants and the medical insurance industry are at an all-time low.

The concept of 'preferred providers' has also been extended to include hospitals and clinics. In more recent years, insurance policies have been linked to networks of hospitals, and a subscriber is only reimbursed if the procedure is carried out in one of these designated hospitals. An exception to this rule will often still be made if a consultant can assure an insurer that a non-network hospital must be used for clinical reasons. These reasons will normally be investigated and must be genuine. As a result, a specialist in a given town can have admission rights to several independent hospitals. This can have an additional advantage in that it can assist him or her to maintain a busy private practice and to be available to all the patients that the GPs in that town and city wish to refer to him or her. The essential network of contacts is, through this means, extended.

The Medical Advisory Committee concept

The Medical Advisory Committee (MAC) concept is playing an increasingly important role in quality assurance and the regulation of standards within the independent hospital sector. Each independent hospital appoints its representative committee of consultant specialists with admission rights. This committee does not have executive powers, but its functions include vetting applicants for admission rights, investigating clinical problems and, in more progressive hospitals, running quality assurance schemes for the reassurance of the public and insurers alike. Committees are normally constitutionally set up and elect a Chairman every year. In addition to ensuring that the specialists with admitting rights are appropriately trained, registered and fulfil the criteria laid down in the legal constitution, good MACs investigate allegations of unsatisfactory medical practice and advise the hospital manager on clinical matters. Increasingly, and although the local MAC has no executive role, it is an unwise hospital manager who makes decisions concerning visiting specialists without discussion and agreement with it. Medical insurance companies can also establish a liaison with local MACs and seek their advice on various matters.

How to antagonise insurance companies

The brief history of the private medical insurance market described above shows its growth and significance in the market for consultants. Most medical insurance businesses have become technically efficient and following the 1992 MMC report, are highly skilled on controlling consultant costs. This may be through crude measures, or through more sophisticated marketing-led concepts, such as 'preferred providers' and 'managed care'.

Successful consultants in private practice have to adapt their businesses to meet the needs of the insurance companies. Those who do not, will, ultimately, lose private practice business. Consultants in practice still commonly commit a number of errors that adversely affect their relationship with their principal direct private income provider. These are listed below.

ERROR 1   Ignore the insurance companies
A small number of consultants in private practice still believes that their income will be generated from overseas patients. Generally this is not so, since it is believed the number of overseas patients being treated in the UK is declining. Most patients are coming from domestic sources with local insurance cover.

ERROR 2   Ignore computerisation
In the late 1990s, claim forms are being electronically transmitted from consultant to insurance company, with payment made electronically directly to his or her bank account. The paper trail is reducing through technical advance. For sheer cost reasons, insurance companies will gravitate towards those consultant practices that are sophisticated electronically and whose systems are compatible. Consultants who ignore office computerisation will be left behind.

ERROR 3   Take time on conducting procedures
Given the interest in cost efficiency, insurance companies are now accumulating a vast array of data on episode costs. For many operations, surgeon costs amount to some 30% of the total, with theatre, drugs, hospital and other costs amounting to a significant 70%. Insurance companies now *know*, for example, which surgeons are more efficient than others in terms of time, cost or procedures. At present, they do not necessarily favour the more efficient surgeon. However, the time is fast approaching, as is commonplace in the USA, when the efficient surgeon will be rewarded financially and the inefficient surgeon penalised.

ERROR 4   Choose the wrong location to run a private practice
The economics of the marketplace call for the most efficient alloca-
tion of resources. Some areas of the country, for example, are
characterised by an ageing or less healthy population, whereas
other areas are characterised by a high proportion of one-parent
families, 'yuppies' and the urban poor. The economics of the
private marketplace inevitably discriminate against the under-
privileged and those who have, in medical terms, a statistically
higher risk of failure. Insurance companies are looking for consultants to be 'successful' and 'efficient'. It follows that those
practising in areas where economic success or medical efficiency is
likely to be below average will earn less from insurance companies
than those conducting their business in more prosperous areas.

ERROR 5   Continue to bundle procedures
As indicated above, this practice is to charge insurance companies
at full price for inter-related procedures which do not in economic
terms, require a separate charge. Through their increasingly
sophisticated databases, insurance companies can now positively
discriminate against consultants engaged in this practice. Not only
are claims being rejected, but, ultimately, consultants can cease to
be recognised.

ERROR 6   Ignore OPCS and insurance company codings
The establishment of large insurance company databases
inevitably involves standardisation to enable more rapid processing of information and speedier processing of payment. There is
still a not insignificant minority of consultants unfamiliar with the
standardised codings required by insurance companies. This is a
function of indiscipline or lack of professionalism. Those consultants who adapt their businesses to cope with insurance company
data requirements can expect more sympathetic consideration in
the longer term.

ERROR 7   Be patient unfriendly
At one time, patients were reluctant to complain to insurance
companies. This is now no longer true, and patients are implicitly
encouraged to complain to insurance companies in cases of poor
service and inattention. Such complaints are investigated, and

persistent consultant offenders may be deregistered. Consultants have increasingly to be conscious of the need to provide a high standard of service in an ambient environment.

ERROR 8   Run an inefficient office
Insurance companies, with their powerful databases, require timely and inefficient input. Some consultants in private practice still run a very inefficient office. Symptoms of this include long delays in replying to correspondence, sloppy attention to insurance company queries, delays in processing claim forms, and general delays and a poor quality of credit control management. Claims managers in insurance companies are inevitably attracted to consultants who operate an efficient service and office, and those who continue to ignore this reality will find themselves increasingly isolated.

ERROR 9   Maintain poor records
The practice of insurance companies independently auditing their providers' records is still in its infancy. Commercial, accounting and quality control pressures are leading to an increase in this activity. Those consultants who maintain a high standard of discipline and accuracy in their patient records will stay on insurance company lists. Those who fail to achieve satisfactory standards will, in time, be removed from insurance company lists as approved suppliers.

ERROR 10   Go into the wrong field of medicine
Sadly, the economics of the marketplace are such that those consultants providing regular, routine and easily quantifiable services will benefit from the rising power of insurance companies. Those whose services are less easily quantifiable (such as, for example, psychologists or psychiatrists) will suffer, income wise. The more wealthy and financially successful consultant will be one who is able to provide consistency, quality and reliability of service in more easily specified procedures. The concept of 'vocation' will, in economic terms, be penalised.

To conclude, the evolving history of the insurance companies has now reached a stage where they dominate the private medical market. Their objectives are to improve efficiency and to control the costs. Those consultants who can embrace these efficiency and quality demands will prosper; those who cannot may find that their practices suffer as a result of loss of status or even recognition by the major financiers.

11

Business planning

The case for business planning

There are two well-known business maxims: that 'organisations do not plan to fail – they fail to plan' and that 'perfect planning prevents poor performance'. Careful planning in business means first, survival, and second, prosperity.

A significant number of young consultants entering private practice for the first time still does not totally accept that they are establishing a new business, which is subject to rules of planning. There is substantial evidence that many in the UK economy who seek to establish their own business fail or, at best, are only partially successful. Failure rates in excess of 50% within two years are not uncommon. Business advisors have long argued that a formal business plan is one of the fundamentals of a successful business. This needs to be realistic. Most business failures in the private medical sector have been, for example, because of unrealistic assumptions about future potential patient numbers.

For an individual consultant formulating a business plan for his or her new private practice, a number of general questions normally need to be considered viz:

- what is your vision for the business?

- what are your *specific* business objectives and targets?

- why do you think that you can achieve these objectives?

- what strategies are you going to employ to achieve these object-ives. In particular, what is the strategy to attract a patient flow?

- what action points are going to be followed to implement these strategies and, of equal importance, what are they going to cost?

- what resources are needed in the business? For example, what consulting room and support space is needed, what communi-cations equipment is required and what staffing is needed (and to what level of training)?

Business and the four 'Ps' of business and marketing planning

The process of marketing is discussed in Chapter 5. From a busi-ness planning perspective, planning for a marketing operation precedes operational implementation. The marketing planning process for a private medical consultant business normally consists of reviewing the so-called 'four Ps of marketing'. These are product, price, promotion and place. In 'product' planning, a number of common questions needs to be addressed:

- what are the market trends that will affect the demand for the service?

- what exactly is the service provided by the consultant?

- what competitive advantage does this service offer over those offered by other consultants?

- who are the competitors?

- what is the appeal in the marketplace to the service?

- does the service offered meet patients' needs?

- how can the product be packaged?

Pricing is the second of the 'four Ps' to be considered in the planning process. Questions concerning the formulation of a pricing policy are considered in Chapter 5. In addition, in the planning process a consultant needs to consider the most effective means of invoicing (credit card, direct settlement, etc.) and for how long, given other market pressures, prices can be maintained.

The third of the 'four Ps' is promotion of service. For a consultant to plan effective promotional activity he or she needs to consider some basic questions:

- what is the target patient market and how is it changing?

- what is the best communication channel to reach this market?

- what are the associated costs?

- what is the precise message that the consultant, in practice, wishes to communicate to potential patients?

- how can this message be effectively communicated?

- is the message clear? Does the consultant overestimate a patient (or even a GP referrer's) intelligence? For the majority of consultants, a brochure is an effective means of promotion directly to the patient. The brochure, coupled with personal presentation, is an important combination to attract GP referrers.

The fourth key 'P' is place. In the business planning process it is not enough to assume that because a consultant is highly skilled surgically or medically, patients will beat a path to the consulting room door. They will not. Although word of mouth is an important factor, other means of communication are important in placing, or distributing, a consultant's message to his or her potential private patients. The successful consultant will need to ensure that he or she has chosen appropriate placement channels. These can include, for example, hospital personnel, GPs or colleagues providing complementary or even computing services.

In considering the most appropriate means of placement of a message, attention does need to be given to the cost of passing information, the training involved, how feedback is handled and how misinformation is handled. New means of distributing a consultant's message need to be reviewed and addressed on a regular basis.

The business plan and, in particular, consideration of the 'four Ps' are now widespread in British business. The science of business planning in the private medical sector is still young. It has been a theme of this book that those who take on board the necessary business disciplines will undoubtedly develop a more successful business than those who believe that medical skills alone are everything. It should be noted that much professional help is available to consultants who believe the process to be too daunting, through specialist accountants, business advisors and local Training and Enterprise Councils.

The SWOT analysis approach

Particularly for those consultants who are daunted by the prospect of an in-depth business planning exercise, there is a simple technique available that has proved to be almost univers-ally successful in generating business planning ideas and in formulating strategies. This is the so-called SWOT analysis approach. Use of this technique involves:

- a frank assessment of the *strengths, weaknesses, opportunities* and *threats* facing a consultant business (the SWOT)
- a systematic review of actions to convert weaknesses into strengths and threats into opportunities
- preparation of an action list
- monitoring of the action list and making revisions where appropriate.

Typically, a consultant's *strengths* are easy to list. These often include:

- his or her technical skills (e.g. the speed and efficiency with which an episode is conducted and the failure rate of procedures)
- the medical sector in which he or she is involved
- the individual personality (e.g. patient friendliness, staff management skills)

- the location of the consultant's practice
- the age of the consultant, which can, in fact, be both a strength and a weakness.

Weaknesses in a consultant's private practice typically include:

- lack of technical skills (e.g. poor technical efficiency, high failure rates on procedures)
- working in an unfashionable medical sector
- a poor personality (e.g. lack of attention to patient care and poor inter-personal and staff management skills)
- poor location of the practice. Some geographical locations are unpopular and unfashionable. Paradoxically, a particular skill is to identify when an unfashionable area suddenly becomes fashionable
- age, particularly if the consultant operates in an area where technology is changing fast.

  It is perhaps a truism that *all* consultants' private practices have *opportunities* to develop. The most frequent opportunities arise from:

  - addressing the impact of changing patient tasks (e.g. for day surgery)
  - taking early advantage of new medical technology, particularly in the areas of procedures and drugs
  - taking advantage of changing methods of delivery of service to patients (e.g. information release, consulting room ambience, 'package deals' and day surgery)
  - relocating as appropriate, to take advantage of the market ebbs and flows of medical skills in the UK.

For those consultants who fail to identify and respond promptly to opportunities available, *threats* to the private practice will become ever dominant. The nature of threats changes over time, but typically includes:

- threat of local and regional competition for consultancy skills

- threat to a private practice of increasingly aggressive insurance company market behaviour

- threat of debilitating illness

- threat of a new technology overwhelming or eliminating demand for an existing medical skill.

For even the smallest of private practices the SWOT analysis is a simple but dynamic business planning tool. Once information is extracted, at any moment in time a consultant or his or her advisor is able to focus on business weaknesses and convert them into strengths. Frequently, the 'action plan' may demand more medical training, investment in facilities and staff, relocation, or training in patient management and care.

The second phase of the SWOT analysis is then to focus carefully on threats and endeavour to convert them to opportunities. Again, a typical action plan will emerge, evolving round training, investment location, marketing and patient management.

The third phase of the SWOT analysis is to set up an interactive and ongoing review process. Practical experience shows that one factor is perhaps more relevant than any other in the use of the SWOT analysis in private medical practice. Most consultants are able to identify their strengths and the opportunities available to them. Many, however, are unable, or reluctant to assess honestly their own weaknesses and the threats facing them. Business honesty and frankness is essential to an effective planning process. The help of other business professionals who can see clearly what an individual sometimes cannot, should always be welcomed.

Specialist planning considerations: the sale of the practice

As they contemplate retirement, many individuals, in all sectors of business, look to sell their business. They hope to generate a profit by selling their business assets and goodwill to others wanting to enter or develop their trade or profession. In the medical sector the value of this practice goodwill to an individual consultant can be quite substantial.

'Goodwill' is a very difficult concept to define. In simple terms it represents the value somebody is prepared to pay for having a stream of patients readily available. It constitutes a payment, as a capital cost, for somebody else's efforts in building up a practice. It is generally accepted that the more successful medical practices have spent many years marketing their services and building up their stream of patients. Such practices may have acquired a significant reputation, whether locally, regionally or nationally.

It is perhaps surprising that in the current climate the market for the sale of private medical practices is still relatively small. There is still a large number of consultants who simply retire, and indeed give away their businesses without seeking to capitalise on past efforts. This situation is in complete contrast to that prevailing in the USA and in other countries, where newly appointed consultants pay to acquire the business of their fellow practitioners who are retiring or contemplating a change in career. Funding from such acquisitions frequently comes from local bankers.

But the market is changing, and the US pattern is likely to follow, with increasing opportunities for sale of practices at a good capital profit. For those consultants who are contemplating a sale of their practice in future, a few well-timed steps are essential.

STEP 1   Maintain a good system of business records
To sell any business effectively, it is important that the record base is sound. For example, full sets of accounts, including business balance sheets for a number of years, lists of patients and their locations, and lists of key contacts or referrers, are essential. Such consultant records should be sufficiently strong to allow for independent audit or verification.

STEP 2   Choose a good advisor
The art of selling any business is specialist. All too often business sales activities are not properly coordinated or managed. As a result, the proceeds achieved by the vendor are less than might otherwise be earned.

STEP 3   Let the advisor 'get on with it'
One of the cardinal sins committed by business vendors is to employ an advisor and then to interfere constantly. A good

advisor will offer the medical consultant a comprehensive service so that he or she can continue with his or her practice without distraction. Such a service will include agreement with the consultant on the optimum time to sell; the research of the market to find potential buyers, such as newly appointed consultants, the detailed valuation of the goodwill and other assets of a consultant's business; the preparation of an appropriate 'practice sale' document, management of the sale process and negotiation with potential practice purchasers; and managing the sale through draft heads of agreement and formal legal documentation.

STEP 4   Keep the sale simple

Given the still immature nature of the market for the sale of consultants' businesses, simplicity is a virtue. In particular, steps should be taken:

• not to be too clever in terms of tax planning

• to try to ensure that a number of individuals are interested in purchase. Healthy competition can often generate a premium

• to try not to seek a firm asking price

• to try to ensure that all matters are totally confidential.

It is true that virtually all consultants in private practice do enjoy some goodwill in their practice, which could be sold if they wish. While the market is undoubtedly changing, it is still strange that a significant number of consultants does not recognise the potential sales value of their practice and does not seek to capitalise on this value at a time of their choosing.

Specialist planning considerations: retirement

Retirement planning, to be effective, should begin early in a consultant's private practice career and should cover a range of factors. In practice, retirement planning exercises conducted by accountants and financial advisors amount to little more than tax planning reviews. These are not necessarily synonymous.

Regular and standard retirement planning advice generally covers four particular aspects.

1. All self-employed consultants and those not in occupational pension schemes should consider maximising their contributions each year to a personal pension plan (PPP) or retirement annuity policy (RAP) up to the limits set by their age and policy. These change each year (Appendix A). For 1998/99, for example, relief is available on earnings up to £87 600 where contributions included payments to a PPP.

2. Consultant members of occupational pension schemes should consider making additional voluntary contributions (AVCs) to the employer's group pension scheme up to a maximum of 15% salary. Contributions have to be paid before 6 April 1999, for example, to qualify for relief in that year.

3. Consultant members of occupational pension schemes nearing retirement need to take specific advice to ensure that the rules enabling a deferral of annuity purchase can be used to maximum effect. Such advice, which is highly technical, can often be better given initially through a professional consultation with a member of the Institute of Actuaries rather than through an independent financial advisor or accountant.

4. Those consultants who are nearing retirement age should consider asking the Department of Social Security for a projection of their state pension entitlement to consider purchasing extra years.

In addition to these steps, a good financial advisor will regularly review a client's 'net relevant earnings' to ensure that there is maximum carry-back of pension payments against prior years. This is to ensure that maximum tax reliefs are available. The rules on pensions are complicated, but careful modelling of a consultant client's affairs can ensure that pensions can be maximised in retirement, and can be effectively used to mitigate his or her tax liability.

A note of caution is needed as a result of the operations of the new self assessment tax system. Maximising pension contributions and simultaneously minimising tax liabilities may not now be possible. Changes in the way tax reliefs are given from April 1997 have caused the Chartered Institute of Taxation to report that a 'substantial proportion' of self-employed people, including consultants, will, from April 1997, probably consistently overpay tax year after year because of the nature of their pension arrangements. Historically consultants have been allowed to 'carry back' pension premiums to previous tax years. Under the new legislation such arrangements and historically efficient tax schemes will be ignored when interim payments for the following tax year are being calculated. The result of these changes is that:

- many consultants will, from January 1999, be paying higher tax bills than they would have done under the 'old' system
- claims for pension relief by then will be deferred.

Medical consultants need to monitor their claims for tax relief to ensure that the forecast of the Chartered Institute of Taxation does not materialise in the long term. However, it may be that for many consultants with both NHS and private income, increasing pension contributions, to be immediately tax efficient, should be made to occupational rather than private pension schemes. Professional advice on the sensitive pensions area is essential at all times.

Retirement planning after the 1998 Budget

The 1998 budget has, with the benefit of very detailed analysis, introduced some major changes to the structure of taxation in the UK. In particular, there are some very significant tax changes that will impact on *all* consultants' retirement strategies.

Consultants approaching 50 years of age should reconsider their retirement strategies now. Those who do can reap the benefit of significant tax concessions and savings. Those who do nothing will have a higher tax burden when they retire than would have been the case prior to April 1998.

The tax changes announced in March 1998 include:

- an increase in the rate of employers' national insurance from 10% to 12.2% from 6 April 1999

- the phasing out of retirement relief for capital gains tax purposes

- the withdrawal of the indexation of capital gains from 6 April 1998

- the introduction of the concept of 'tapering' considering a capital gain

- the abolition of advanced corporation tax from 6 April 1999

- the reduction in the rate of corporation tax on small companies from 21% to 20% from 6 April 1999.

These changes, when taken in concert, will lead to fundamental changes in the tax climate facing all medical consultants when planning retirement. Steps that should be taken within three years from 6 April 1998 include:

- review of retirement planning strategy

- a review of pensions planning

- for those consultants approaching 50 years of age immediate decisions as to whether to 'retire' for tax purposes

- consideration of the merits of trading as a small company. The tax treatment of small companies appears to be increasingly favourable

- consideration of the merits of incorporating a consultant's private practice, thereby reducing potential capital gains tax liabilities, while at the same time reducing the overall tax burden.

Following the 1998 Budget, the opportunities for a consultant in private practice to plan for his or her retirement in a tax efficient way have perhaps never been greater. Certainly the differentials for 'getting it right' and 'getting it wrong' have, after April 1998, never been wider. 'Getting it right' for a sophisticated consultant businessman can reduce average tax liabilities to under 30% on retirement. 'Getting it wrong' can increase tax liability by nearly 200% of what would have been paid prior to April 1998. Careful professional assessment of a consultant's business, of his or her motivations and objectives, and a thorough detailed knowledge of the implications of the 1998 tax changes are essential to the financially and commercially aware consultant. For most consultants, a professional consultation now will be an investment that can reap high dividends.

Specialist planning considerations: divorce

It is currently estimated that the national divorce rate in the UK is in excess of 40%. Informal estimates suggest that for those in the medical profession the proportion is higher, probably in the 50–55% range. The reasons for this higher divorce rate are not hard to find: the stress of a rapidly changing profession and of working in the NHS or private practice; long hours spent at work which are incompatible with the needs of family life; the breaking of the traditional family network; changing financial circumstances and the regular opportunity to meet new partners.

Any sensible businessman faced with the prospect of a risk greater than 50% would undoubtedly take steps to mitigate the potential loss. It is therefore not totally illogical to suggest that those medical consultants in private practice should plan financially for a divorce.

For those consultants unfortunate enough to go through divorce proceedings, the financial consequences can be catastrophic. Apart from the heavy legal costs (which in reality benefit neither party financially), there are many unforeseen costs and expenses. All of these add to the emotional trauma of a divorce. Accountants are frequently involved in the financial unscrambling of consultants' marriages. Sensible planning by both parties can reduce something of the financial pain. Practical experience shows that planning can reduce damage.

TIP 1   Be frank at the outset
It is much easier if consultants and their partners are aware of each other's financial position at the outset of a marriage. With this information both parties can plan priorities and avoid risks of claims of deceit if troubles arise.

TIP 2   Don't rush financial divorce
Careful analysis, including assessment of pension rights, can often lead to a more equitable, stable, long-term arrangement than ill-thought-out rapid financial separation.

TIP 3   Stop spending
Once a consultant's relationship has broken down, bitter experience has shown that it is often important to close all joint accounts, credit cards, loans, overdrafts and hire purchase arrangements as soon as possible.

TIP 4   Protect both parties' interests in the family home
Homes are commonly owned by partners either as 'joint' or 'beneficial' joint tenants. As a first step in the event of an irretrievable breakdown, the couple should agree to a 'beneficial joint tenant' arrangement to protect their individual interests. In this way, in the event of a death, sole interest does not revert to the survivor.

TIP 5   Be honest
At times of marital breakdown, mutual trust and respect often decline rapidly. Either party may be tempted not to disclose assets or attempt to dispose of these in a way unbeknown to their partners. Angry partners have been known to 'whistle blow' on consultants, for example, who regularly accept cash from their patients, thereby triggering a serious tax investigation.

TIP 6   Seek financial advice
Experience has shown that taking impartial independent advice at an emotionally charged time can benefit a consultant and his or her partner.

TIP 7   Find an appropriate lawyer
It is not unknown for lawyers to stimulate acrimony to increase their fees. To minimise disruption to a consultant's business and life, it is important to identify a sympathetic, commercially sensible lawyer who can stand above and not foster acrimony, and, above all, who can achieve results.

TIP 8   Take legal advice
The legal aspects of divorce are complex. Specialist divorce lawyers often have the additional skills needed to achieve objectives rapidly.

TIP 9   Try conciliation
Experience has shown that those medical consultants who have been able to tackle difficult issues through mediation and counselling have often found a solution more satisfactory to both themselves and their partners.

TIP 10   Keep your spirits up
The stress of divorce affects medical practitioners as much as anybody else. History includes examples of individual surgeons or clinicians unable to face their patients or even unable to operate as a result of ongoing personal pressures. It is important that consultants keep their spirits up because their professional responsibilities and skills are still required. Patients have no interest in a consultant's private problems and neither should they. In such difficult times, the strong personal support of friends and colleagues is often essential merely to keep going.

Divorce is a feature of medical life. History provides examples of sound medical practices that have failed because of the immense personal and financial pressures of a divorce. A recognition of this risk, coupled with sound planning, can reduce the potential impact of what is a tragic personal event.

12

Future developments and adjustments to change

There is a maxim that states that in 100 years' time the world will be full of new people. In this current fast-changing environment perhaps a more appropriate maxim would be to say that in 10 years' time the world will be full of new consultants!

The only certain factor in a modern consultant's business life is a level of uncertainty. The picture of Mr Cox, the medical consultant in 2010, perhaps typifies what is to come.

The working consultant in 2010: prophesy or fantasy?

Mr Cox was one of the few private consultants left working in Harley Street in 2010. For some years, the street had been the centre of a multitude of companies and franchise operations providing medical and insurance services. The many bistros, restaurants and flowers shops on the street catered for the smart-suited accountants and marketing executives who now effectively ran the medical profession.

Mr Cox reflected on the last year of the NHS as he knew it in 2003. Most of the country's hospitals had been sold off to the multi-national insurance companies. General practice doctors' businesses had been taken over by various franchise groups who charged a royalty fee for management services and marketing.

For a couple of years after that, until 2005, the old NHS accident and emergency service had remained as a state-financed operation. Tax payers were each given a voucher entitling them to services from the rump of the NHS up to a strict cash limit. The system proved costly to a country which had finally run out of its oil reserves and the NHS 'Accident and Emergency plc' was first regionalised and subsequently sold off to a series of independent bidders. The Health Regulators Office continued to this day to supervise the performance of the Accident and Emergency companies and dealt with some of the worst excesses of companies pursuing a profit motive to the exclusion of all else.

Mr Cox remembered the days when managing his business affairs was relatively easy. The medical sector had, of course, been fully incorporated into the Value Added Tax regime since the 2001 Budget and he had now to complete his monthly returns. These were fully integrated with his tax returns. Self assessment had become ever more sophisticated and formal, with clever Treasury ministers devising a means whereby all self-employed people accounted for tax on their earnings on a monthly basis, as did employees. The electronic billing systems to patients and from insurers did take care of the paperwork, though checking figures to ensure accuracy and to avoid very heavy fines for error remained a bore.

Mr Cox's first appointment of the day was with his public relations agent. Surgeons had, since the turn of the century, been subject to heavy litigation for even minor errors. A vast legal sector had grown in recent years specialising in health litigation. To cover the constant claims and rising insurance premiums, most young surgeons had joined the insurance companies and worked exclusively at their hospitals. Those older surgeons remaining needed the assistance of public relations agents in their dealings with the media and with their own patients.

The second appointment was with Mr Cox's marketing manager. Marketing was important. Mr Cox found it difficult to fix prices in the ever-competitive market. Following the Monopolies and Mergers Commission report into price fixing by the leading insurance companies in 2004, and the subsequent banning of benefit scales, there were absolutely no data available by which prices could be compiled. In addition to pricing, Mr Cox had tried every marketing device to attract patients – package deals, loyalty points and free gifts. He was now looking at a new scheme pioneered as long ago as the 1990s: introduce a friend and help yourself to a free gift. Mr Cox was sure that this would increase his patient numbers.

The operation programme began after these two key meetings, which took up most of the morning. Mr Cox had operations planned for Belfast, Newcastle and Birmingham that day. His three television screens had been set up by his personal assistant. He checked with the operating theatre in Belfast. All was ready and he moved over to his console. He punched in the commands and the robot in Belfast took over. He pressed a button and watched progress on a giant screen at the side. Regular Technicolor photographs and print-outs emerged from the printer. These would be used for patient records and for assisting in reprograming the robot. Mr Cox thought of the times when those in medical practice did not even have to take a first degree in computer science and robotics.

One hour later, the operations were complete and Mr Cox's assistant pressed the keyboard to ensure the processing of electronic fee notes and the transfer of funds to his account. His assistant prepared a copy of the operations documents for submission to the Medical Defence Union official who religiously collected the files each day for checking. How strange, he thought, that the mandatory checking programme of each procedure was not carried out electronically. Mr Cox closed the computer down, after checking his own computer's rating index on his performance. What would medicine be like, he thought, in 10 years' time when he would be enjoying his retirement?

The business factors likely to change a consultant's business

A large number of factors that impact on a private consultants' practice is already in process of change. Some of the more important changes are listed below.

Continuing uncertainty and frustration in the NHS

It is likely that the NHS will continue to evolve. Financial restrictions will inevitably continue, with the services focusing increasingly on accident and emergency and more sophisticated medical work. There appears to be no end in sight to the ongoing sense of frustration felt by many. Nonetheless, the NHS will continue to form the bedrock of career development for most consultants and the prime basis for their contact network.

Increasing role of insurance companies

It is likely that insurance companies will continue to maintain pressure on fees charged by their providers. Cost management under a variety of guises will continue. In addition, quality control and audit of consultants' services are likely to become more sophisticated.

Ongoing technological change

The pace of technological change shows no sign of abatement. The pressures on consultants to master and acquire new techniques, and for an ongoing programme of re-education and supplementary education are likely to continue.

Changes in private practice business conduct and performance

While there will be changes in the NHS, in technology and in the role of insurance companies, the conduct and management of private practices will change. Principal changes are likely to be:

- the increasing regionalisation of private practice

- the development of franchising and groupings of consultants with particular specialties

- the increasing rate of medical litigation as Britain follows the US model

- the increased role of professional marketing to a successful medical practice

- increasing emphasis on quantitative analysis for consultants' performances and patient information. This may be under the guise of 'best practice' or 'quality management' but more openness appears a certainty

- the increasing note of direct patient advertising. There appear to be signs that the traditional role of the GP as a prime referrer may be breaking down. Historically, GPs have tended to refer private patients to those consultants who have serviced them well in the NHS. In future, a specialist's reputation is more likely to be made by a marketing man than the NHS or personal contact with GPs. The more successful consultants are likely to be those of whom the public has heard.

While the impact of these and other factors on his or her business will vary, a consultant in practice will continue to trade in uncertain waters. There is no certainty to his or her business life. In this respect, a private medical consultant's future shows no change from that which it has always been, or to the climate facing any business. Those who face the challenge of change will survive. Those who cannot will have to find other careers.

It is hoped that some of the suggestions in this book will help medical consultants in private practice cope with the business changes facing them and take maximum advantage of the opportunities that change brings.

Appendix A
Tax facts 1998–99

A. Income tax

Rate of tax	Taxable income	
	1998–99	1997–98
	£	£
Lower rate 20%	0–4300	0–4100
Basic rate 23%	4301–27 100	4101–26 100
Higher rate 40%	over 27 100	over 26 100

20% on dividends and savings income if not liable to higher rate.

Main personal allowances	1998–99	1997–98
	£	£
Personal	4195	4045
Married couple's (a) (b)	1900	1830
Age allowance (age on 5.4.99)		
Age 65–74		
Personal	5410	5220
Married couple's (a) (b)	3305	3185

Age 75 or over		
Personal	5600	5400
Married couple's (a) (b)	3345	3225
Income limit for age allowances	16 200	15 600
Additional personal (a)	1900	1830
Blind person's	1330	1280
Widow's bereavement (a)	1900	1830

(a) Relief given at 15% (15%) only.
(b) Claimed by husband, but on election, £1900 (£1830) may be claimed by wife or shared equally. Transferable on election if insufficient income.

Mortgage interest relief

Relief at 10% (15%) on qualifying loans up to a maximum of £30 000 (£30 000).

B. Car benefits

1998–99 (and 1997–98)

Business mileage per annum		Percentage of list price (a)	
First car	Second car	Under 4 years old at 5.4.99	4 or more years old at 5.4.99
Under 2500	Under 18 000	35%	23.3%
2500–17 999	18 000 or more	23.33%	15.56%
18 000 or more		11.67%	7.78%

(a) Includes certain accessories, but reduced for capital contributions of up to £5000 (£5000). The upper limit including accessories is fixed at £80 000.

Fuel benefit	1998–99		1997–98	
	Petrol £	Diesel £	Petrol £	Diesel £
Engine capacity				
Up to 1400 cc	1010	1280	800	740
1401–2000 cc	1280	1280	1010	740

| More than 2000 cc | 1890 | 1890 | 1490 | 940 |
| Cars without a cylinder | 1890 | | 1490 | |

Fixed profit car scheme

The authorised mileage rates which apply for business mileage in the year 1998–99 (unchanged from 1997–98) are shown in the table below.

Engine capacity	On the first 4000 miles in the tax year	On each mile over 4000 miles in the tax year
Up to 1000 cc	28p	17p
1001c–1500 cc	35p	20p
1501–2000 cc	45p	25p
over 2000 cc	63p	36p

C. Inheritance tax

Threshold: 1998–99, £223 000; 1997–98, £215 000. A flat rate of tax of 40% is levied for transfers in excess of the threshold. For transfers made within seven years of death a reduced charge applies.

Years between death and gift	0–3	3–4	4–5	5–6	6–7
Percentage of death rate (%)	100	80	60	40	20

D. Personal pensions (PPs) and retirement annuities (RAPs)

Age on 6 April	% of net relevant earnings	
	RAP	PP
35 or less	17.5	17.5
36–45	17.5	20.0
46–50	17.5	25.0
51–55	20.0	30.0

	1998–99	1997–98
56–60	22.5	35.0
61–74	27.5	40.0

Earnings cap	1998–99	1997–98
	£87 600	£84 000

E. Capital gains tax

Rate

As if gains were top slice of individual's income. Trusts generally 34%.

	1998–99 £	1997–98 £
Annual exemption	6800	6500
Trusts generally	3400	3250
Personal representatives for year of death and next two years only	6800	6500

Indexation relief frozen at April 1998. Chargeable gains then reduced by reference to period of ownership post-April 1998. Abatement of 75% for business assets held 10 years tapering to 7.5% for 1 year. Abatement of 40% for non-business assets held 10 years tapering to 5% for 3 years' ownership.

F. National insurance contributions

From 6 April 1998

Class 1 – Individuals in employment

Lower earnings limit (LEL) £64 weekly, £278 monthly, £3328 yearly. There is no liability for either employees' or employers' contributions if earnings are below these limits.

Upper earnings limit (UEL) £485 weekly, £2102 monthly, £25 220 yearly. Applies to employees only.

	Employee		Employer
Standard rate if weekly earnings above LEL	First £64	Balance	On all earnings
£64 to £109.99	2%	10%	3%
£110 to £154.99	2%	10%	5%
£155 to £209.99	2%	10%	7%
£210 to £485	2%	10%	10%
Over £485	no additional liability		10%

	First		First	
Contracted-out rate if weekly earnings above LEL	£64	Balance	£64	Balance
£64 to £109.99	2%	8.4%	3%	NIL
£110 to £154.99	2%	8.4%	5%	2%
£155 to £209.99	2%	8.4%	7%	4%
£210 to £485	2%	8.4%	10%	7%
Over £485	no additional liability		10%	above rate up liability to £485 excess 10%

Employer contributions (contracted-out): rates above are for salary-related schemes. For money-purchase schemes rates are 1.5% higher on weekly earnings between £64 and £485.

Class 2 – Self-employed individuals

£6.35 per week. Earnings under £3590 per annum are exempt.

Class 3 – Voluntary contributions

£6.25 per week.

Class 4 – Self-employed individuals

6% on assessable profits between £7310 and £25 220 a year.

G. Corporation tax

	Financial year to	
	31.3.99	31.3.98
Main rate	31%	31%
Small companies rate	21%	21%
Lower limit	£300 000	£300 000
Upper limit	£1.5m	£1.5m
Effective rate on marginal profits	33.5%	33.5%
Rate of ACT	1/4	1/4

H. Value added tax

	From 1.4.98	From 1.12.97
Standard rate	17.5%	17.5%
Registration level	£50 000	£49 000
De-registration level	£48 000	£47 000

I. Stamp duty

Stamp duty on sales	From 24.3.98	To 23.3.98
Stocks and shares	0.5%	0.5%
Other property (rate applies to whole price)		
£0–£60 000	Nil%	Nil%
£60 001–£250 000	1%	1%
£250 001–£500 000	2%	1.5%
£500 001 or more	3%	2%
Stamp duty reserve tax	0.5%	0.5%

All figures are calculated inclusive of VAT, if any.

J. Savings

Personal Equity Plans

General PEP limit	£6000
Single company limit	£3000
Unit and investment trust limit	£6000
Non-EC unit and investment trust limit	£6000

Tax-Exempt Special Savings Account

Maximum Year 1	£3000
Maximum Year 2–4	£1800
Maximum investment over 5 years	£9000
Re-investment into second generation TESSA	£9000

Note: From 6.4.99 new TESSA and PEP accounts will not be available as tax free investments and will now come under the new ISA scheme.

K. Capital allowances

Machinery and plant		
– normal rate	25%	reducing balance
– first year allowance *	50%	to 1 July 1998 (12% for certain long-life assets **)
	40%	from 2 July 1998
– long-life assets **	6%	reducing balance
Motor cars	25%	reducing balance (maximum £3000 pa)
Industrial buildings and qualifying hotels	4%	of cost per annum
Commercial or industrial buildings in an enterprise zone	100%	
Agricultural buildings	4%	of cost per annum
Scientific research	100%	
Know-how	25%	reducing balance
Patient rights	25%	reducing balance

* Applies to small and medium-sized businesses (as defined by the Companies Act). Cars and certain other assets are excluded.

** Assets with a working life of 25 years or more unless expenditure on such assets is below £100 000 in the period.

L. Key dates

Self assessment

31 July 1998	Second 1997/98 payment on account for all taxpayers.

30 September 1998	Tax return deadline if the Inland Revenue is to calculate tax liability for 1997/98.
	Deadline for notifying new sources of income.
31 January 1999	Final deadline for submitting tax returns. Balance of 1997/98 tax liability and first payment on account for 1998/99 due.

Inheritance tax

Death: normally 6 months after month of death.
Lifetime transfer 6 April–30 September: 30 April in following year.
Lifetime transfer 1 October–5 April: 6 months after month of transfer.

Corporation tax

Pay and file: 9 months after accounting period.

Advance corporation tax

Normally 14 days after 31 March, 30 June, 30 September, 31 December and accounting year end.

Subject to Finance Act 1998.

Appendix B
Private medical practice legal audit: typical documentation review content

(NOTE: Not all documents are appropriate to, or required by, a given private medical practice. Each review will be based on the business structure.)

1. Employment

Service contracts
Statement of terms of employment
Employment contracts
Disciplinary and grievance procedures
Trade unions
Health and safety
Professional assistants
Contractors
Employee share options (where trading as a limited company)
Other
Note: Most consultants with an NHS contract should also seek to have this reviewed.

2. Business documents

Sale documents
Purchase documents
Terms of business
Sale conditions
Purchase conditions
Business name strategy
Joint ventures
Agents
Distributors (where appropriate)
Franchise (where appropriate)
Other

3. Licences

Consumer Credit Act
Financial Services Act
Data Protection Act
Licensing Act
Gaming Act
Other

4. Property

Leasehold
Freehold
Planning consents
Planning agreements
Other

5. Intellectual property

Patents
Copyright

Trade/Service marks
Registered design
Other

6. Insurance

Property
Public
Product
Keyman
Buyout
Director's liability (for those trading as companies)
Professional indemnity and negligence
Other

7. Pensions

Business pensions
Trust deeds
Rules
Periodic report
Superannuation fund
Directors' personal pensions (for those trading as companies)
Other

8. Trade and professional associations

Rules
Recommendations
Codes
Other

9. Medical and other equipment

Hire

Hire purchase
Lease
Lease/Sale
Other

10. Computer

Hardware agreement
Maintenance
Software licence
Software maintenance
Bureau
Escrow deposit
Other

11. Litigation and credit control

Claims

12. Partnership

For those practising as a partnership

Agreement
Other partnership considerations

13. Constitution

For those practising through a limited company

Memorandum
Articles
Amending resolutions
Shareholders' agreements
Statutory books (see Section 16)
Minute books

Accounts and returns
Other

14. Shareholders and finance

Shares/Stock
Mortgage/Charges
Debentures
Loans (also for other forms of private practice organisations)
Personal guarantees/Indemnity (also for other forms of private
   practice organisations)
Bonds
Bank facility (also for other forms of private practice organisations)
Sale and leaseback
Other

15. Company forms

The legislation stresses the need to ensure standard information is
available for all companies. Failure to file forms by any company
many result in:

- a criminal penalty where time limits are exceeded

- a civil penalty for late filing of accounts

- some actions being declared illegal

- notification before action in some cases

16. Statutory records

Every company is required to keep:

- register of members

- register of charges

- register of directors and secretaries

- register of directors' interests
- directors' service contracts
- minute books (board and general)
- register of substantial interests in voting shares (plcs only)
- accounting records

Index

Appendix B
Private medical practice legal audit: typical documentation review content

(NOTE: Not all documents are appropriate to, or required by, a given private medical practice. Each review will be based on the business structure.)

1. Employment

Service contracts
Statement of terms of employment
Employment contracts
Disciplinary and grievance procedures
Trade unions
Health and safety
Professional assistants
Contractors
Employee share options (where trading as a limited company)
Other
Note: Most consultants with an NHS contract should also seek to have this reviewed.

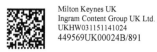

9 781857 752236